The Comprehensive Diabetic Diet
Cookbook for Beginners

1500- Day Easy & Flavorful Recipes to Combat Prediabetes and Type 2 Diabetes without Sacrificing Taste, Along with a 28-Day Meal Plan

Maureen J. Britton

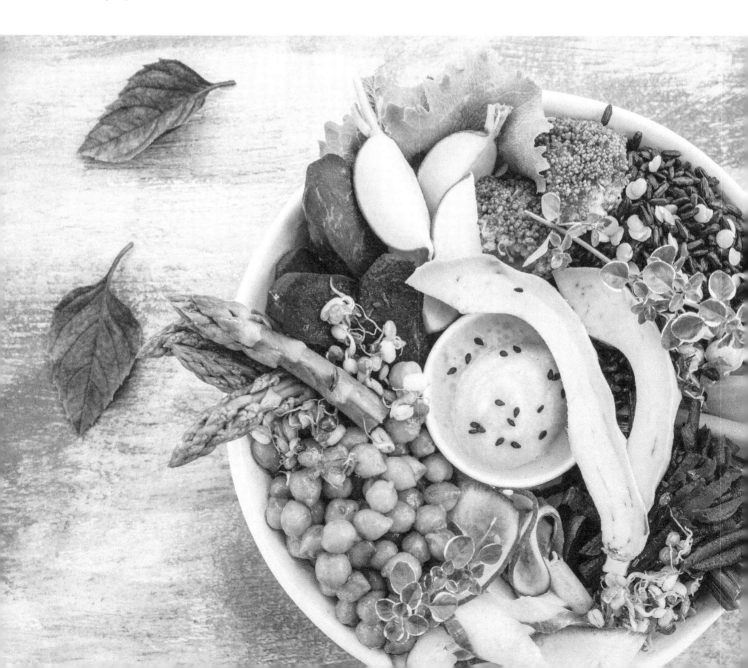

Table of Contents

Chapter 3 Beans and Grains 28

Chapter 4 Beef, Pork, and Lamb 35

Chapter 5 Poultry 46

Chapter 6 Fish and Seafood 57

Chapter 7 Snacks and Appetizers 66

Chapter 8 Vegetables and Sides 73

Chapter 9 Vegetarian Mains   82

Chapter 10 Stews and Soups   91

Chapter 12 Salads   106

Appendix 1: Measurement Conversion Chart   116

Appendix 2: The Dirty Dozen and Clean Fifteen   117

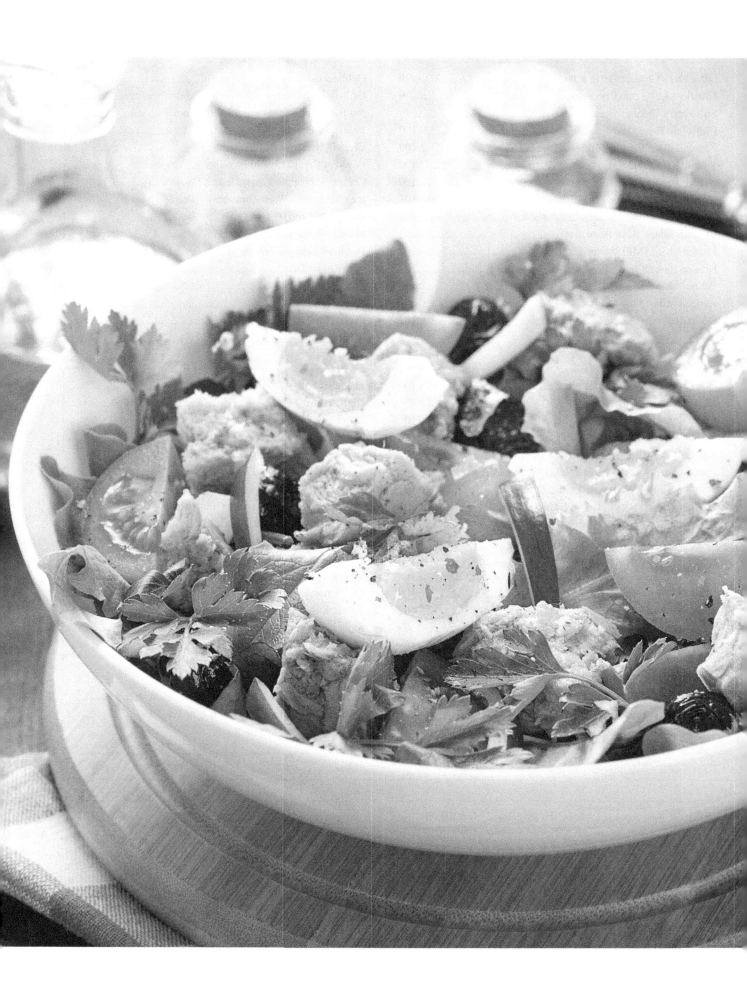

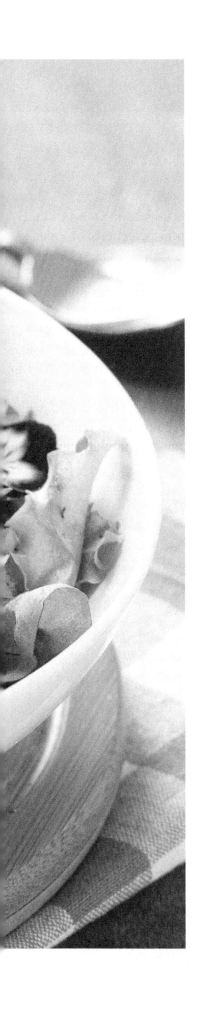

INTRODUCTION

Welcome to the world of diabetic cookbook. I am thrilled to have you join me on this culinary journey designed specifically for individuals with diabetes. My purpose is simple yet powerful: to provide you with a wide array of delicious and nutritious recipes that will support your health goals while satisfying your taste buds.

Living with diabetes can present its unique challenges, and I understand the importance of maintaining a balanced diet to effectively manage blood sugar levels. That's why I have carefully curated each recipe in this cookbook to strike the perfect balance between taste, nutrition, and blood sugar management. I want to dispel the misconception that a diabetic diet has to be restrictive or dull. With this cookbook, you can indulge in flavorful meals while taking control of your health.

I recognize the adjustments and conscious choices we individuals with diabetes face every day. Managing diabetes can sometimes feel overwhelming, but I am here to support you. My aim is to simplify the process by providing practical recipes and helpful tips that can be easily incorporated into your daily routine. I want you to feel empowered and confident in your ability to create meals that are not only healthy but also incredibly satisfying.

This cookbook is your companion on the journey to managing diabetes through the power of food. My goal is to show you that eating well with diabetes is both achievable and enjoyable. I want these recipes to not only nourish your body but also nurture your spirit, reminding you that taking care of yourself can be a joyful and delicious experience.

As you embark on this culinary adventure, I encourage you to embrace the journey of self-care through food. See cooking and eating as opportunities for self-expression, creativity, and nourishment. Discover new flavors, experiment with ingredients, and tailor recipes to your personal taste preferences. Let this cookbook be a source of inspiration and a platform for you to share your experiences, modifications, and discoveries with our community of readers.

Together, let's celebrate the joy of nourishment and the pleasures of the table. Get ready to experience a world of diabetic delights that will make managing your health an enjoyable and flavorful endeavor.

Chapter 1 Diabetic Diet

Understanding of Diabetes and Diet

Living with diabetes requires a thorough understanding of the condition and its impact on your health. By gaining knowledge about diabetes and its relationship with diet, you can make informed choices to manage your blood sugar levels effectively.

Diabetes is a chronic condition that affects the body's ability to regulate blood sugar, either due to insufficient insulin production or ineffective use of insulin. It is important to recognize that diet plays a vital role in managing diabetes alongside medication and other treatment strategies.

To effectively manage diabetes through diet, it is crucial to understand the significance of portion control and the selection of appropriate ingredients. Portion control helps regulate the intake of carbohydrates, which have the most significant impact on blood sugar levels. By managing portion sizes, you can avoid spikes in blood sugar and maintain stable levels throughout the day.

Controlling portion sizes involves being mindful of the quantity of food consumed and learning to gauge appropriate servings. It can be helpful to measure portions initially until you become more familiar with visual cues. Additionally, paying attention to hunger and satiety cues can guide you in determining appropriate portion sizes for your individual needs.

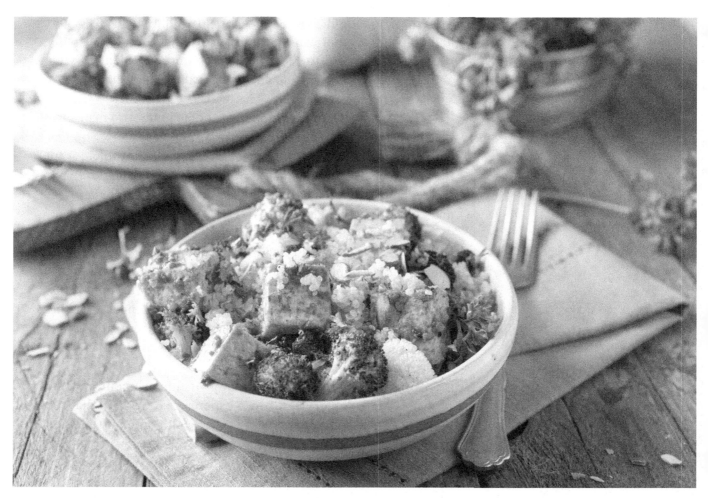

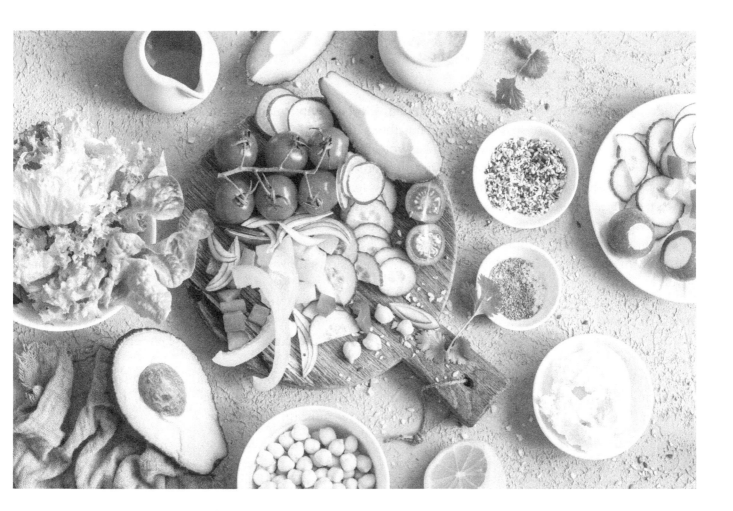

Choosing the right ingredients is equally important. Opting for foods that are low in added sugars and unhealthy fats helps maintain steady blood sugar levels and supports overall health. Emphasizing whole, unprocessed foods like fruits, vegetables, lean proteins, and whole grains provides essential nutrients while minimizing the risk of blood sugar fluctuations.

Fruits and vegetables are excellent choices for their high fiber content, which aids in slowing down the absorption of carbohydrates and promoting better blood sugar control. When selecting carbohydrates, prioritize complex carbohydrates such as whole grains, legumes, and starchy vegetables over refined options. These complex carbohydrates offer more fiber, vitamins, and minerals, providing sustained energy and better blood sugar management.

Incorporating lean proteins, such as poultry, fish, tofu, and beans, into your meals helps stabilize blood sugar levels and promotes satiety. These protein sources also offer essential nutrients while being lower in unhealthy fats compared to their higher-fat counterparts.

It is equally important to be mindful of fat intake. Choosing healthier fats, such as avocados, nuts, seeds, and olive oil, provides essential fatty acids while minimizing the risk of cardiovascular complications associated with diabetes.

By grasping these fundamental concepts of portion control and ingredient selection, you can lay a solid foundation for managing your diabetes effectively through your diet.

In the upcoming sections of this cookbook, I will provide practical tips and guidance on diabetes-friendly cooking. These suggestions will empower you to make smart choices when it comes to selecting and preparing ingredients, managing portion sizes, and adapting recipes to suit your needs.

Together, we will navigate the intricate relationship between diabetes and diet, ensuring that you have the knowledge and tools to make delicious, healthy choices that support your well-being. Let's embark on this journey of understanding and discover the immense potential of food as a powerful ally in managing diabetes.

Practical Tips for Diabetes-Friendly Cooking

Preparing diabetes-friendly meals doesn't have to be complicated or restrictive. With a few practical tips and strategies, you can create delicious and nutritious dishes that support your blood sugar management goals. Here are some key pointers to keep in mind as you embark on your diabetes-friendly cooking journey:

♦ Choose wholesome ingredients: Opt for whole, unprocessed foods as the foundation of your meals. These include fresh fruits, vegetables, whole grains, lean proteins, and legumes. These nutrient-dense choices provide essential vitamins, minerals, and dietary fiber while minimizing added sugars and unhealthy fats.

♦ Mindful carbohydrate selection: Carbohydrates have the most significant impact on blood sugar levels. Focus on incorporating complex carbohydrates, such as whole grains (e.g., quinoa, brown rice, whole wheat), into your meals. These choices offer more fiber, which slows down digestion and helps stabilize blood sugar levels.

♦ Portion control: Be mindful of portion sizes to manage your carbohydrate intake effectively. Use measuring cups, a food scale, or visual cues to gauge appropriate portions. Balancing your plate with non-starchy vegetables, lean protein, and healthy fats in addition to carbohydrates can help create satisfying and balanced meals.

♦ Incorporate lean proteins: Lean proteins play a crucial role in managing blood sugar levels and promoting satiety. Include sources such as skinless poultry, fish, tofu, legumes, and low-fat dairy products. These options offer high-quality protein without excessive unhealthy fats.

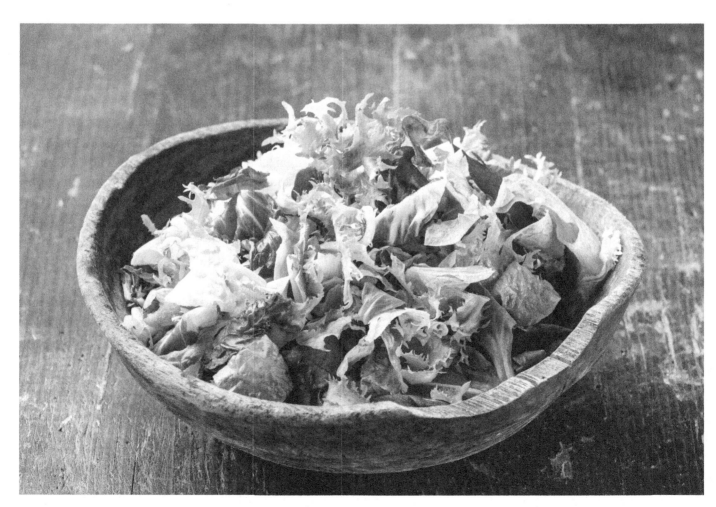

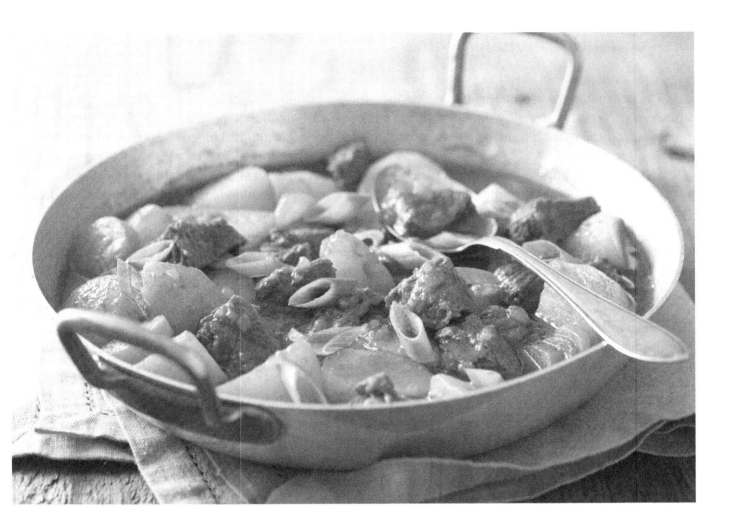

♦ Healthy cooking methods: Choose cooking methods that minimize the need for added fats and promote healthier outcomes. Opt for grilling, baking, steaming, or sautéing with minimal oil instead of deep-frying or pan-frying. These methods help retain the natural flavors of the ingredients while reducing the overall calorie and fat content of the dish.

♦ Flavor with herbs and spices: Enhance the taste of your meals without relying on excessive salt, sugar, or unhealthy fats. Experiment with a variety of herbs, spices, and citrus juices to add depth and complexity to your dishes. This way, you can enjoy flavorful meals while reducing the need for less healthy additives.

♦ Healthy fats in moderation: While it's important to limit unhealthy fats, incorporating healthy fats in moderation can be beneficial. Include sources like avocados, nuts, seeds, and olive oil. These options provide essential fatty acids and can contribute to a satisfying and well-balanced meal.

♦ Stay hydrated: Don't forget the importance of staying hydrated. Water should be your primary beverage of choice. Limit or avoid sugary drinks, including soda and fruit juices, as they can cause blood sugar spikes.

♦ Meal planning and preparation: Planning your meals in advance can help you make healthier choices and avoid impulsive decisions. Set aside time for meal prep, batch cooking, or pre-cutting ingredients to make cooking more convenient and manageable throughout the week.

♦ Consult a healthcare professional: Every individual's dietary needs may vary. It's essential to consult with a registered dietitian or healthcare professional who specializes in diabetes management to develop a personalized meal plan that meets your specific requirements.

By implementing these practical tips, you can navigate the world of diabetes-friendly cooking with confidence. Remember, small changes in your cooking and eating habits can make a significant difference in managing your blood sugar levels effectively and enjoying delicious meals at the same time.

Essential Nutritional Information

Understanding the essential nutrients and their impact on blood sugar levels is key to managing diabetes effectively. By familiarizing yourself with the basics of carbohydrates, proteins, fats, fiber, vitamins, and minerals, you can make informed choices to support your overall health and blood sugar control.

1. Carbohydrates:

Carbohydrates are the macronutrients that have the most significant impact on blood sugar levels. When consumed, they break down into glucose, leading to an increase in blood sugar. It's important to focus on the type and quantity of carbohydrates in your diet. Complex carbohydrates, such as whole grains, legumes, and vegetables, are digested more slowly, causing a gradual rise in blood sugar. On the other hand, simple carbohydrates, found in processed and sugary foods, can lead to rapid spikes in blood sugar. Monitoring your carbohydrate intake and choosing healthier sources is crucial for maintaining stable blood sugar levels.

2. Proteins:

Proteins play a crucial role in repairing and building body tissues. They have a minimal impact on blood sugar levels and can help promote satiety and stabilize energy levels. Lean protein sources, such as skinless poultry, fish, tofu, beans, and low-fat dairy products, are excellent choices. Be mindful of portion sizes and aim to include protein in each meal to support overall health and blood sugar management.

3. Fats:

Fats provide energy, aid in the absorption of fat-soluble vitamins, and contribute to the flavor and texture of foods. While it's important to moderate fat intake to maintain a healthy weight, not all fats are created equal. Healthy fats, such as monounsaturated and polyunsaturated fats found in avocados, nuts, seeds, and olive oil, have been associated with improved heart health and better blood sugar control. Limit saturated fats and avoid trans fats, commonly found in fried and processed foods, as they can increase the risk of heart disease and worsen insulin resistance.

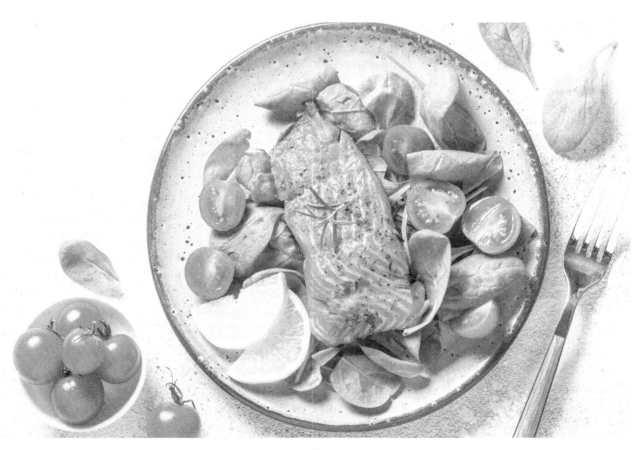

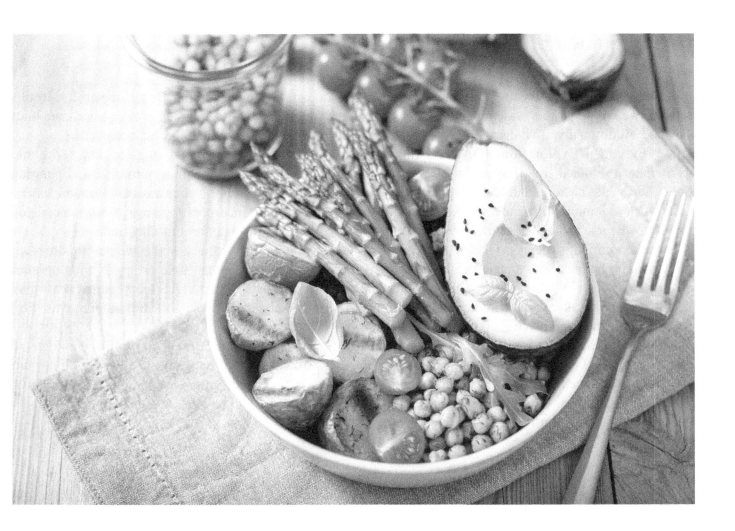

4. Fiber:

Dietary fiber is a type of carbohydrate that the body cannot digest. It plays a vital role in promoting digestive health, controlling blood sugar levels, and maintaining a healthy weight. There are two types of fiber: soluble and insoluble. Soluble fiber, found in foods like oats, legumes, and fruits, forms a gel-like substance in the digestive system, slowing down the absorption of glucose and helping to stabilize blood sugar levels. Insoluble fiber, found in whole grains and vegetables, adds bulk to the stool, aiding in regular bowel movements.

5. Vitamins and Minerals:

A balanced diet rich in fruits, vegetables, whole grains, and lean proteins provides a wide array of essential vitamins and minerals. These micronutrients play critical roles in supporting overall health and helping the body function optimally. While there is no specific vitamin or mineral that directly lowers blood sugar levels, deficiencies in certain nutrients can impact insulin function and overall metabolic health. It is important to consume a varied and nutrient-dense diet to meet your body's needs.

By understanding the role of carbohydrates, proteins, fats, fiber, vitamins, and minerals, you can make educated choices when planning your meals. Creating a well-rounded and balanced diet that includes a variety of nutrient-rich foods will not only help manage blood sugar levels but also promote overall health and well-being. Remember to consult with a healthcare professional or registered dietitian for personalized guidance on incorporating essential nutrients into your diabetes management plan.

Explore a Variety of Flavors and Adaptations

Creating delicious meals while managing diabetes doesn't mean sacrificing flavor or variety. In this section, we will explore a wide range of flavors, ingredients, and cooking techniques to keep your taste buds satisfied. Additionally, we'll discuss ways to adapt recipes to suit your dietary preferences and needs.

♦ Flavorful Explorations: Discover the world of spices, herbs, and seasonings to add depth and excitement to your dishes. Experiment with aromatic spices like cinnamon, cumin, turmeric, and paprika. Fresh herbs like basil, cilantro, mint, and rosemary can elevate the flavors of your meals. Citrus juices and zests, such as lemon, lime, and orange, provide a burst of freshness. By incorporating a variety of flavors, you can enjoy diverse and delicious meals without relying on excessive salt, sugar, or unhealthy fats.

♦ Customizing Recipes: One of the joys of cooking is the ability to customize recipes to suit your individual preferences and dietary needs. Whether you prefer vegetarian, gluten-free, or low-sodium options, adapting recipes is a way to ensure they align with your health goals. Swap ingredients, adjust seasoning levels, or explore alternative cooking methods to create dishes that cater to your specific requirements. Feel free to get creative and make each recipe your own!

♦ Balancing Macronutrients: When modifying recipes, it's important to maintain a balance of macronutrients. Focus on incorporating lean proteins, complex carbohydrates, and healthy fats into your meals. This balance helps provide sustained energy, promotes satiety, and supports stable blood sugar levels. By making mindful ingredient substitutions and portion adjustments, you can create meals that are not only delicious but also supportive of your overall health.

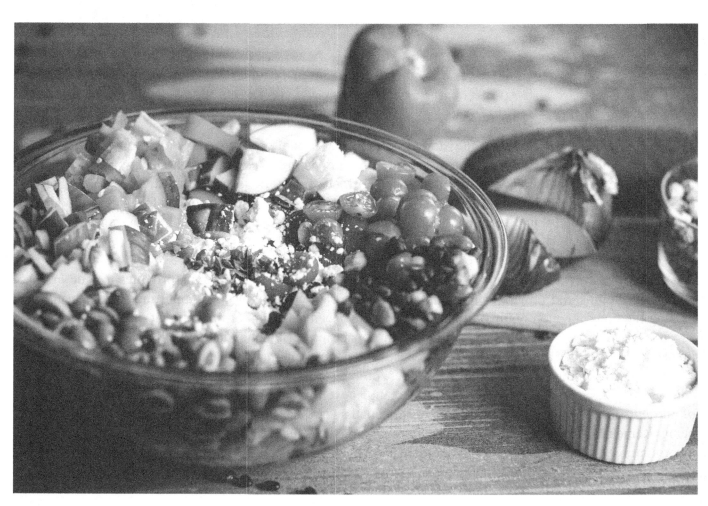

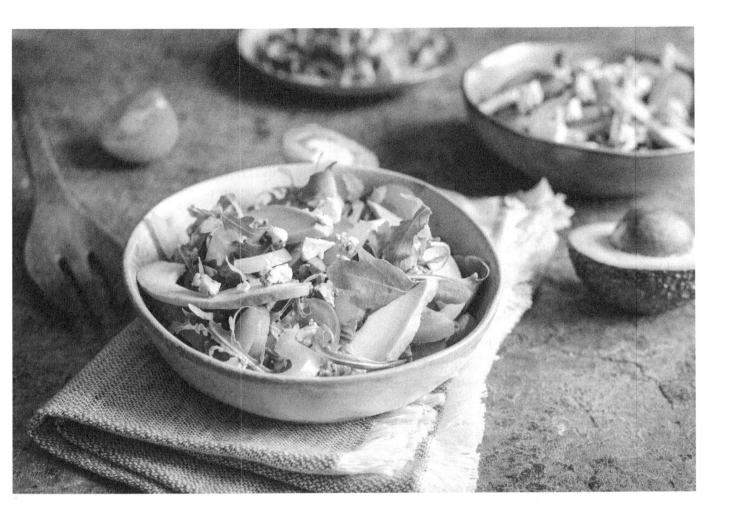

♦ Diverse Meal Options: Embrace the opportunity to explore various meal categories, including breakfast, appetizers, main dishes, side dishes, snacks, and desserts. Each category offers a plethora of possibilities for creating diabetes-friendly and enjoyable meals. Incorporate a variety of fruits, vegetables, whole grains, and lean proteins into your daily menu to ensure a well-rounded and balanced diet.

♦ Engaging with the Community: Don't forget the power of community and shared experiences. Connect with other individuals managing diabetes to exchange recipe ideas, cooking tips, and support. Online forums, cooking groups, and social media communities can provide valuable insights and inspiration for your culinary journey. Sharing your own adaptations and successes can also help inspire others and foster a sense of camaraderie.

Remember, cooking is a creative and personal process. Use these guidelines to explore new flavors, adapt recipes to your preferences, and create meals that nourish both your body and soul. The possibilities are endless, and by embracing experimentation and enjoying the process, you'll discover a world of culinary delights that are perfectly suited to your diabetes management plan.

Mastering Cooking Techniques and Utilizing Essential Tools

To become a confident and skilled cook while managing diabetes, it's essential to familiarize yourself with various cooking techniques and utilize the right tools. By understanding how different methods affect flavors, textures, and nutritional profiles, you can create wholesome and delicious meals. Let's delve into some cooking techniques and tools that will enhance your culinary prowess.

1. Sautéing and Stir-Frying:

Sautéing and stir-frying are excellent techniques for quickly cooking ingredients while preserving their flavors and nutrients. Use a non-stick pan or a small amount of heart-healthy oil to lightly coat the surface. By keeping the heat high and continuously stirring or tossing the ingredients, you can achieve a vibrant, crisp texture without excessive oil absorption.

2. Roasting and Baking:

Roasting and baking are versatile techniques that add depth and richness to your meals. By using dry heat in the oven, you can enhance flavors and achieve desirable textures. Roasting vegetables brings out their natural sweetness, while baking proteins like chicken or fish helps retain moisture. Both methods require minimal oil, making them ideal for healthy cooking.

3. Grilling and Broiling:

Grilling and broiling provide a distinct smoky flavor and caramelization to your dishes. Grilling involves cooking over an open flame or hot grill, while broiling utilizes direct heat from the oven's top element. These techniques are perfect for cooking lean proteins, vegetables, and fruits, adding a delicious charred touch without the need for excessive fats.

4. Steaming:

Steaming is a gentle and healthy cooking method that retains the nutrients and natural flavors of ingredients. It involves cooking food over boiling water, either in a steamer basket or wrapped in foil or parchment paper. Steaming is particularly suitable for vegetables, fish, and delicate proteins. It requires no additional fat and helps maintain the food's texture and color.

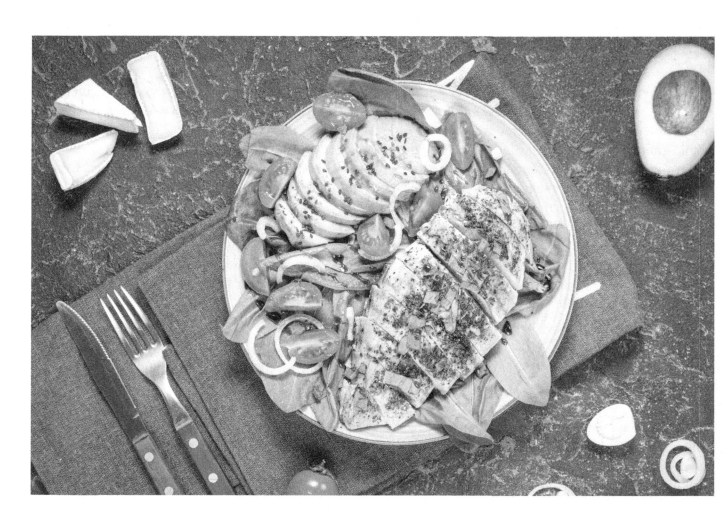

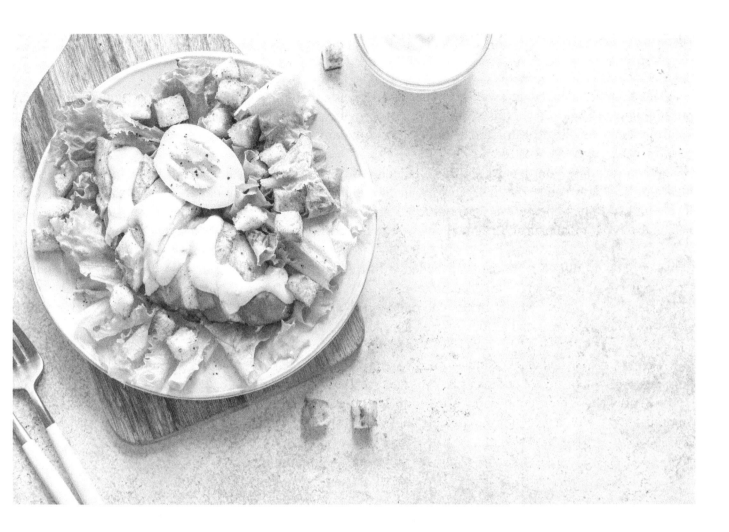

5. Slow Cooking:

Slow cooking is a convenient and time-saving technique that allows flavors to meld and intensify over long periods. It involves cooking ingredients at low temperatures for an extended time, usually in a slow cooker or a Dutch oven. This method is ideal for soups, stews, and braised dishes, as it tenderizes tougher cuts of meat and allows for easy batch cooking.

6. Essential Kitchen Tools:

Equipping your kitchen with essential tools can streamline your cooking process and ensure optimal results. Some indispensable items include:

♦ A sharp chef's knife for precise cutting and chopping.
♦ Cutting boards for a clean and organized workspace.
♦ Non-stick pans or skillets for healthier cooking with minimal oil.
♦ Baking sheets and pans for roasting and baking.
♦ Steamer baskets or inserts for gentle and nutritious steaming.
♦ Slow cookers or Dutch ovens for convenient slow cooking.
♦ Measuring cups and spoons for accurate portion control.
♦ Kitchen scales for precise ingredient measurement.
♦ Blender or food processor for smoothies, sauces, and purees.
♦ Grilling tools like tongs, brushes, and skewers for outdoor or indoor grilling.

By mastering various cooking techniques and utilizing essential tools, you'll be well-equipped to create a wide range of delicious and diabetes-friendly meals. Remember to prioritize techniques that require minimal added fats, emphasize natural flavors, and preserve the nutritional integrity of your ingredients. With practice and curiosity, you'll gain confidence in the kitchen and create meals that are both nourishing and satisfying.

Sample Meal Plans and Portion Guidance

Developing balanced and well-portioned meal plans is a fundamental aspect of managing diabetes and promoting overall health. In this section, we will provide sample meal plans and offer guidance on portion control to help you create a structured approach to your daily meals.

1. Meal Planning Basics:

When planning your meals, aim for a balance of carbohydrates, proteins, and fats while incorporating plenty of vegetables and fruits. Distribute your food intake throughout the day to support stable blood sugar levels and sustained energy. It's essential to consult with a healthcare professional or registered dietitian to personalize your meal plan according to your specific needs, medications, and lifestyle.

2. Sample Meal Plan - Breakfast:

♦ Option 1: Whole-grain oatmeal topped with fresh berries, a sprinkle of nuts, and a drizzle of honey. Enjoy a side of Greek yogurt for added protein.

♦ Option 2: Veggie omelet made with egg whites, spinach, mushrooms, and bell peppers. Serve with a slice of whole-grain toast and a side of sliced avocado.

3. Sample Meal Plan - Lunch:

♦ Option 1: Grilled chicken breast salad with mixed greens, cherry tomatoes, cucumber, and a vinaigrette dressing. Pair with a side of quinoa or brown rice.

♦ Option 2: Whole-grain wrap filled with lean turkey or tofu, fresh vegetables, and a light spread of hummus. Serve with a side of raw vegetable sticks and a small portion of fruit.

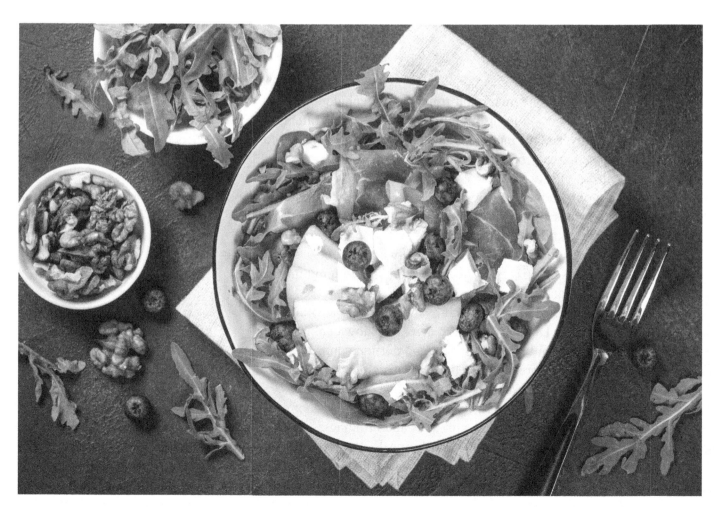

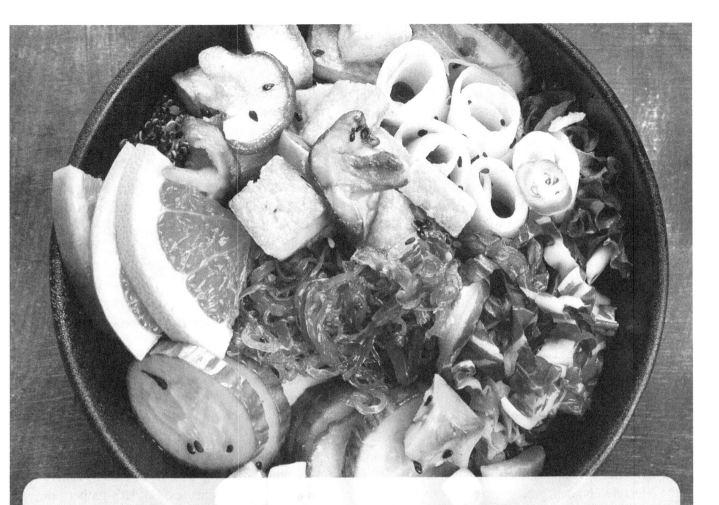

4. Sample Meal Plan - Dinner:

♦ Option 1: Baked salmon fillet with a lemon-dill sauce, served alongside steamed asparagus and quinoa pilaf.

♦ Option 2: Grilled chicken or tofu stir-fry with a colorful mix of bell peppers, broccoli, carrots, and snap peas. Use a light soy sauce or low-sodium teriyaki sauce for flavor. Serve over brown rice or cauliflower rice.

5. Sample Meal Plan - Snacks:

Option 1: A small handful of mixed nuts and seeds.

Option 2: Greek yogurt with sliced fruits or a small apple with a tablespoon of nut butter.

Option 3: Raw vegetable sticks with hummus or a hard-boiled egg.

6. Portion Control:

Maintaining portion control is crucial for managing blood sugar levels and maintaining a healthy weight. Here are some general guidelines:

♦ Carbohydrates: Aim for about 45-60 grams of carbohydrates per meal. This can vary depending on your individual needs and goals. Use measuring cups or a food scale to portion out grains, fruits, and starchy vegetables.

♦ Proteins: Include a palm-sized portion (about 3-4 ounces) of lean protein, such as skinless poultry, fish, tofu, or legumes, in each main meal.

♦ Fats: Limit added fats and use them sparingly. Aim for about 1-2 tablespoons of healthy fats, like olive oil, avocado, or nuts, per meal.

♦ Vegetables: Fill half of your plate with non-starchy vegetables, such as leafy greens, broccoli, cauliflower, zucchini, and peppers. These nutrient-dense options provide fiber and essential vitamins and minerals.

Remember, these sample meal plans and portion guidelines are meant to provide a starting point and should be adjusted to suit your individual needs and preferences. It's important to work with a healthcare professional or registered dietitian who can help create a personalized meal plan that considers your specific health goals, medications, and dietary requirements.

In conclusion, I extend a warm welcome to you as you embark on this culinary journey through the pages of this diabetic cookbook. My purpose in creating this cookbook is to empower individuals like you, who are managing diabetes, to take control of their health and well-being through the art of mindful and delicious cooking.

Within these pages, you will find a wealth of knowledge and practical guidance. Together, we will explore the intricate relationship between diabetes and diet, understanding the impact of various nutrients on blood sugar levels and overall health. Through the sharing of essential nutritional information, you will gain insights into the role of carbohydrates, proteins, fats, fiber, vitamins, and minerals in managing your diabetes effectively.

I am excited to share practical tips for diabetes-friendly cooking, enabling you to confidently navigate your kitchen and create flavorful dishes that align with your dietary preferences. You will discover how to harness the power of diverse flavors, experiment with spices and herbs, and adapt recipes to suit your unique tastes and needs.

Furthermore, we will delve into the mastery of cooking techniques and the utilization of essential tools, equipping you with the skills and knowledge needed to create wholesome meals that nourish both your body and soul. With the inclusion of sample meal plans and portion guidance, you will have a structured approach to your daily meals, while still allowing room for customization and personalization.

Together, we embark on a journey of wellness and culinary delight. Through the exploration of delicious recipes, the discovery of new flavors, and the understanding of how to make positive lifestyle choices, you will be empowered to thrive in managing your diabetes. So, let's gather our ingredients, don our aprons, and begin this exciting culinary adventure together.

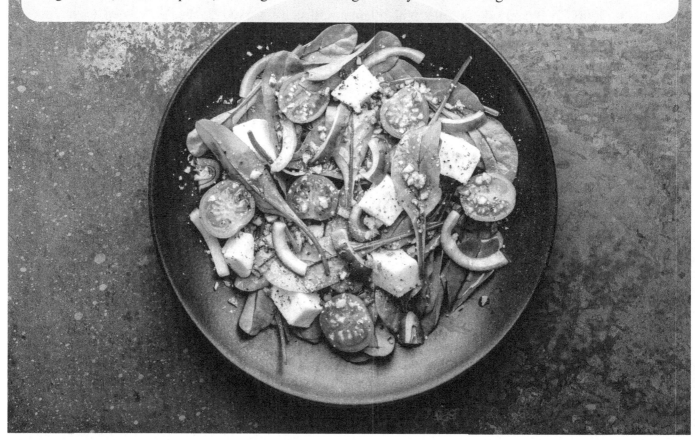

28 Days Diabetic Diet Meal Plan

DAYS	BREAKFAST	LUNCH	DINNER	SNACK/DESSERT
1	Tropical Greek Yogurt Bowl	Zucchini Ribbons with Tarragon	Goat Cheese-Stuffed Flank Steak	Pomegranate–Tequila Sunrise Jelly Shots
2	Avocado Toast With Tomato And Cottage Cheese	Dijon Roast Cabbage	Italian Zucchini Boats	Chocolate Baked Bananas
3	Instant Pot Hard-Boiled Eggs	Simple Bibimbap	Chickpea "Tuna" Salad	Mango Nice Cream
4	Spicy Tomato Smoothie	Mushroom Cassoulets	Three Bean and Basil Salad	Strawberry Cream Cheese Crepes
5	Italian Frittata	Parmesan-Rosemary Radishes	Power Salad	Pineapple Pear Medley
6	Green Eggs and Ham	Best Brown Rice	Winter Chicken and Citrus Salad	Grilled Watermelon with Avocado Mousse
7	Overnight Berry Oats	Green Beans with Garlic and Onion	Lentil Salad	Walnut Macaroons
8	Pumpkin Apple Waffles	Teriyaki Chickpeas	Warm Sweet Potato and Black Bean Salad	Chipotle Black Bean Brownies
9	Shredded Potato Omelet	Garlicky Cabbage and Collard Greens	Salmon Niçoise Salad	Strawberry Cheesecake in a Jar
10	Southwestern Egg Casserole	Moreish Lemony Quinoa	Chickpea Salad	Crustless Key Lime Cheesecake
11	Cinnamon Wisp Pancakes	Caramelized Onions	Shrimp Peri-Peri	Avocado Chocolate Mousse
12	Creamy Green Smoothie	Summer Squash Casserole	Lemon-Basil Turkey Breasts	Orange Praline with Yogurt
13	Broccoli-Mushroom Frittata	Brussels Sprouts with Pecans and Gorgonzola	Mediterranean Chef Salad	Broiled Pineapple
14	Cocoa Carrot Muffins	Lemon-Garlic Mushrooms	Rainbow Quinoa Salad	Simple Bread Pudding
15	Golden Potato Cakes	Horseradish Mashed Cauliflower	Cucumber-Mango Salad	Chewy Chocolate-Oat Bars
16	Veggie And Egg White Scramble With Pepper Jack Cheese	Soft-Baked Tamari TofuSauce	Grilled Romaine with White Beans	Ambrosia

DAYS	BREAKFAST	LUNCH	DINNER	SNACK/DESSERT
17	Pumpkin Spice Muffins	Pico de Gallo Navy Beans	Cabbage Slaw Salad	Cream Cheese Swirl Brownies
18	Mi-So Love Avocado Toast	Spicy Mustard Greens	Shanghai Salad	Low-Fat Cream Cheese Frosting
19	Avocado-Tofu Scramble with Roasted Potatoes	Garlic Herb Radishes	Chicken Reuben Bake	No-Bake Chocolate Peanut Butter Cookies
20	Cauliflower Scramblel	Zucchini on the Half Shell	Roast Chicken with Pine Nuts and Fennel	Double-Ginger Cookies
21	Berry–French Toast Stratas	Sherried Peppers with Bean Sprouts	Herbed Tomato Salad	Oatmeal Cookies
22	Oat and Walnut Granola	Cauliflower with Lime Juice	Chicken, Cantaloupe, Kale, and Almond Salad	Cream Cheese Shortbread Cookies
23	Buckwheat Crêpes with Fruit and Yogurt	Roasted Eggplant	Young Kale and Cabbage Salad with Toasted Peanuts	Creamy Pineapple-Pecan Dessert Squares
24	Seedy Muesli	Smashed Cucumber Salad	Triple-Berry and Jicama Spinach Salad	Banana Pineapple Freeze
25	White Bean–Oat Waffles	Sun-Dried Tomato Brussels Sprouts	Wild Rice Salad	Instant Pot Tapioca
26	Pumpkin Walnut Smoothie Bowl	Sweet-and-Sour Cabbage Slaw	Blueberry and Chicken Salad on a Bed of Greens	Ice Cream with Warm Strawberry Rhubarb Sauce
27	Bran Apple Muffins	Broiled Asparagus	Herbed Spring Peas	Spiced Pear Applesauce
28	Eggplant Breakfast Sandwich	Garlic Roasted Broccoli	Strawberry-Spinach Salad	Oatmeal Raisin Cookies

Chapter 2 Breakfasts

Breakfast Hash

Prep time: 10 minutes | Cook time: 30 minutes |
Serves 6

Oil, for spraying
3 medium russet potatoes, diced
½ yellow onion, diced
1 green bell pepper, seeded and diced

2 tablespoons olive oil
2 teaspoons granulated garlic
1 teaspoon salt
½ teaspoon freshly ground black pepper

1. Line the air fryer basket with parchment and spray lightly with oil. 2. In a large bowl, mix together the potatoes, onion, bell pepper, and olive oil. 3. Add the garlic, salt, and black pepper and stir until evenly coated. 4. Transfer the mixture to the prepared basket. 5. Air fry at 400ºF (204ºC) for 20 to 30 minutes, shaking or stirring every 10 minutes, until browned and crispy. If you spray the potatoes with a little oil each time you stir, they will get even crispier.

Per Serving:

calories: 133 | fat: 5g | protein: 3g | carbs: 21g | fiber: 2g | sodium: 395mg

Cauliflower Scramble

Prep time: 5 minutes | Cook time: 5 minutes | Serves 3

1 package (12 to 16 ounces) medium or medium-firm tofu
3½ to 4 cups steamed cauliflower florets, lightly mashed
½ teaspoon onion powder
½ teaspoon garlic powder
½ teaspoon sea salt

¼ teaspoon prepared mustard
½ teaspoon black salt (or another ¼ teaspoon sea salt)
½ tablespoon tahini
2½ to 3 tablespoons nutritional yeast
2 to 3 cups chopped spinach or kale

1. In a large nonstick skillet, use your fingers to crumble the tofu, breaking it up well. Place the skillet over medium heat. Add the cauliflower, onion powder, garlic powder, sea salt, mustard, and black salt. Cook for 3 to 4 minutes, then add the tahini and nutritional yeast and stir to combine thoroughly. If the mixture is sticking, add 1 to 2 tablespoons water. Add the spinach or kale during the final minutes of cooking, stirring until just nicely wilted and still bright green. Taste, season as desired, and serve.

Per Serving:

calorie: 196 | fat: 9g | protein: 21g | carbs: 16g | sugars: 3g | fiber: 10g | sodium: 862mg

Green Eggs and Ham

Prep time: 5 minutes | Cook time: 10 minutes |
Serves 2

1 large Hass avocado, halved and pitted
2 thin slices ham
2 large eggs
2 tablespoons chopped green onions, plus more for garnish

½ teaspoon fine sea salt
¼ teaspoon ground black pepper
¼ cup shredded Cheddar cheese (omit for dairy-free)

1. Preheat the air fryer to 400ºF (204ºC). 2. Place a slice of ham into the cavity of each avocado half. Crack an egg on top of the ham, then sprinkle on the green onions, salt, and pepper. 3. Place the avocado halves in the air fryer cut side up and air fry for 10 minutes, or until the egg is cooked to your desired doneness. Top with the cheese (if using) and air fry for 30 seconds more, or until the cheese is melted. Garnish with chopped green onions. 4. Best served fresh. Store extras in an airtight container in the fridge for up to 4 days. Reheat in a preheated 350ºF (177ºC) air fryer for a few minutes, until warmed through.

Per Serving:

calories: 316 | fat: 25g | protein: 16g | carbs: 10g | sugars: 1g | fiber: 7g | sodium: 660mg

Seedy Muesli

Prep time: 5 minutes | Cook time: 0 minutes | Makes
6 cups

2 cups gluten-free rolled oats
1 cup roasted, slivered almonds
¾ cup raw sunflower seeds
½ cup raw pumpkin seeds
½ cup pistachios

½ cup apricots, sliced
¼ cup hemp seeds
¼ cup ground flaxseed
¼ cup toasted sesame seeds

1. In a medium bowl, combine the oats, almonds, sunflower seeds, pumpkin seeds, pistachios, apricots, hemp seeds, flaxseed, and sesame seeds. 2. Store the mixture in an airtight container at room temperature for up to 6 months.

Per Serving:

1 cup: calories: 494 | fat: 36g | protein: 23g | carbs: 38g | sugars: 5g | fiber: 14g | sodium: 9mg

Brussels Sprouts and Egg Scramble

Prep time: 5 minutes | Cook time: 20 minutes | Serves 4

Avocado oil cooking spray
4 slices low-sodium turkey bacon
20 Brussels sprouts, halved

lengthwise
8 large eggs
¼ cup crumbled feta, for garnish

1. Heat a large skillet over medium heat. When hot, coat the cooking surface with cooking spray and cook the bacon to your liking. 2. Carefully remove the bacon from the pan and set it on a plate lined with a paper towel to drain and cool. 3. Place the Brussels sprouts in the skillet cut-side down, and cook for 3 minutes. 4. Reduce the heat to medium-low. Flip the Brussels sprouts, move them to one side of the skillet, and cover. Cook for another 3 minutes. 5. Uncover. Cook the eggs to over-medium alongside the Brussels sprouts, or to your liking. 6. Crumble the bacon once it has cooled. 7. Divide the Brussels sprouts into 4 portions and top each portion with one-quarter of the crumbled bacon and 2 eggs. Add 1 tablespoon of feta to each portion.

Per Serving:

calories: 314 | fat: 22g | protein: 20g | carbs: 10g | sugars: 3g | fiber: 4g | sodium: 373mg

Cocoa Carrot Muffins

Prep time: 5 minutes | Cook time: 23 to 24 minutes | Makes 12 muffins

2 cups spelt flour (or 1¾ cups whole wheat pastry flour)
⅓ cup coconut sugar
¼ cup cocoa powder
1 teaspoon cinnamon
½ teaspoon nutmeg
¼ teaspoon sea salt
2 teaspoons baking powder
½ teaspoon baking soda
2 tablespoons nut butter, such

as almond or cashew butter (or 1½ tablespoons tahini mixed with 1 tablespoon maple syrup)
1 cup low-fat nondairy milk
¾ cup unsweetened applesauce
1 cup grated carrot
¼ cup raisins
2 tablespoons sugar-free nondairy chocolate chips (optional)

1. Preheat the oven to 350°F. Line a muffin pan with 12 parchment cupcake liners. 2. In a large bowl, combine the flour, sugar, cocoa, cinnamon, nutmeg, salt, baking powder, and baking soda, stirring well. In a medium bowl, combine the nut butter with a few tablespoons of the milk, whisking it to incorporate fully. Continue to add the remaining milk and then the applesauce, stirring thoroughly. Add this wet mixture to the dry, along with the carrot, raisins, and chips (if using). Fold and mix until just combined; do not overmix. Spoon the batter into the cupcake liners. Bake for 23 to 24 minutes, or until a toothpick inserted in the center comes out clean. Remove from the oven, let cool in the pan for a couple of minutes, then transfer to a cooling rack.

Per Serving:

1 muffin: calorie: 137 | fat: 2g | protein: 4g | carbs: 28g | sugars: 11g | fiber: 4g | sodium: 205mg

Mi-So Love Avocado Toast

Prep time: 5 minutes | Cook time: 2 minutes | Serves 1

2 slices sprouted grain bread
1 to 1½ teaspoons chickpea miso (or other mild-flavored miso)
¼ cup ripe avocado, mashed
Squeeze of lemon juice (about ½ teaspoon)
A couple pinches of sea salt

1 teaspoon nutritional yeast (optional)
Freshly ground black pepper to taste
2 thick slices ripe tomato, or a handful of chopped lettuce or baby spinach

1. Toast the bread. While it's still warm, spread about ½ teaspoon of the miso on each slice. Distribute the avocado over the miso, and add a squeeze of lemon juice and a pinch of salt. Sprinkle on nutritional yeast (if using), and pepper. Top with the sliced tomatoes, lettuce, or spinach.

Per Serving:

calorie: 250 | fat: 8g | protein: 7g | carbs: 38g | sugars: 4g | fiber: 6g | sodium: 1190mg

Avocado-Tofu Scramble with Roasted Potatoes

Prep time: 5 minutes | Cook time: 25 minutes | Serves 4

1½ pounds small potatoes, cut into bite-size pieces
4 tablespoons plant-based oil (safflower, olive, or grapeseed), divided
Kosher salt
Freshly ground black pepper
1 ounce water
2 teaspoons ground cumin

2 teaspoons turmeric
¼ teaspoon paprika
1 yellow onion, finely chopped
1 bell pepper, finely chopped
3 cups kale, torn into bite-size pieces
3 ounces firm tofu, drained and crumbled
1 avocado, diced, for garnish

1. Preheat the oven to 425°F. Line a baking sheet with parchment paper. 2. Combine the potatoes with 2 tablespoons of oil and a pinch each of salt and pepper on the baking sheet, then toss them to coat. Roast for 20 to 25 minutes or until tender and golden brown. 3. Meanwhile, stir together the water, cumin, turmeric, and paprika until well mixed to make the sauce. Set aside. 4. Heat the remaining 2 tablespoons of oil in a large skillet over medium heat. Add the onion and bell pepper and sauté for 3 to 5 minutes. Season with a pinch of salt and pepper. 5. Add the kale to the skillet, cover, and allow the steam to cook the kale for about 2 minutes. 6. Remove the lid and, using a spatula, push the vegetables to one side of the skillet and place the tofu and sauce on the empty side. Stir until the tofu is heated through, 3 to 5 minutes. Stir the tofu and vegetables. 7. Serve the tofu scramble with the roasted potatoes on the side and garnished with avocado.

Per Serving:

calories: 385 | fat: 23g | protein: 8g | carbs: 42g | sugars: 3g | fiber: 9g | sodium: 25mg

Spicy Tomato Smoothie

Prep time: 5 minutes | Cook time: 0 minutes | Serves 2

1 cup tomato juice	Juice of 1 lemon
2 tomatoes, diced	1 teaspoon hot sauce
¼ English cucumber	4 ice cubes

1. Put the tomato juice, tomatoes, cucumber, lemon juice, hot sauce, and ice cubes in a blender and blend until smooth. 2. Pour into two glasses and serve.

Per Serving:

calories: 51 | fat: 1g | protein: 2g | carbs: 11g | sugars: 7g | fiber: 2g | sodium: 34mg

Italian Frittata

Prep time: 10 minutes | Cook time: 30 minutes | Serves 6

2 tablespoons extra-virgin olive oil	2 teaspoons garlic, minced
2 medium yellow onions, sliced thinly	1 bunch fresh basil, finely chopped
6 large eggs, beaten until foamy	½ teaspoon freshly ground black pepper
2 cups mixed steamed vegetables (try chopped broccoli, asparagus, and red bell peppers)	¼ cup freshly grated Parmigiano-Reggiano cheese, for garnish

1. Preheat the oven to 350 degrees. Add the oil to a large, wide, ovenproof skillet and heat over medium heat. 2. Add the onions and sauté until lightly golden, approximately 5–10 minutes. 3. In a large bowl, combine the remaining ingredients (except the cheese), and add to the skillet. 4. Place the skillet in the oven and bake the frittata for 14–17 minutes until set. Remove from the oven and loosen the edges with a spatula. Sprinkle with grated cheese, cut into wedges, and serve.

Per Serving:

calories: 160 | fat: 11g | protein: g9 | carbs: 8g | sugars: 3g | fiber: 2g | sodium: 159mg

Overnight Berry Oats

Prep time: 5 minutes | Cook time: 0 minutes | Serves 2

1 cup rolled oats	nondairy milk (plus more for serving, if desired)
1 cup raspberries or mixed berries (such as blueberries, strawberries, and blackberries), fresh or frozen	½ tablespoon chia seeds
1 cup + 1–2 tablespoons low-fat	2 tablespoons coconut nectar or pure maple syrup
	Pinch of sea salt

1. In a bowl or large jar, combine the oats, berries, milk, chia seeds,

nectar or syrup, and salt. Cover and refrigerate overnight (or for at least several hours). Serve with more milk to thin, if desired, and also try some additional add-ins.

Per Serving:

calorie: 326 | fat: 5g | protein: 9g | carbs: 64g | sugars: 21g | fiber: 14g | sodium: 205mg

Simple Buckwheat Porridge

Prep time: 5 minutes | Cook time: 40 minutes |
Serves 4

2 cups raw buckwheat groats	1 cup unsweetened almond milk
3 cups water	
Pinch sea salt	

1. Put the buckwheat groats, water, and salt in a medium saucepan over medium-high heat. 2. Bring the mixture to a boil, then reduce the heat to low. 3. Cook until most of the water is absorbed, about 20 minutes. Stir in the milk and cook until very soft, about 15 minutes. 4. Serve the porridge with your favorite toppings such as chopped nuts, sliced banana, or fresh berries.

Per Serving:

calories: 314 | fat: 3g | protein: 10g | carbs: 67g | sugars: 5g | fiber: 9g | sodium: 52mg

Shredded Potato Omelet

Prep time: 15 minutes | Cook time: 20 minutes |
Serves 6

3 slices bacon, cooked and crumbled	¼ cup fat-free milk
2 cups shredded cooked potatoes	¼ teaspoon salt
	⅛ teaspoon black pepper
¼ cup minced onion	1 cup 75%-less-fat shredded cheddar cheese
¼ cup minced green bell pepper	1 cup water
1 cup egg substitute	

1. With nonstick cooking spray, spray the inside of a round baking dish that will fit in your Instant Pot inner pot. 2. Sprinkle the bacon, potatoes, onion, and bell pepper around the bottom of the baking dish. 3. Mix together the egg substitute, milk, salt, and pepper in mixing bowl. Pour over potato mixture. 4. Top with cheese. 5. Add water, place the steaming rack into the bottom of the inner pot and then place the round baking dish on top. 6. Close the lid and secure to the locking position. Be sure the vent is turned to sealing. Set for 20 minutes on Manual at high pressure. 7. Let the pressure release naturally. 8. Carefully remove the baking dish with the handles of the steaming rack and allow to stand 10 minutes before cutting and serving.

Per Serving:

calories: 130 | fat: 3g | protein: 12g | carbs: 13g | sugars: 2g | fiber: 2g | sodium: 415mg

Summer Veggie Scramble

Prep time: 10 minutes | Cook time: 10 minutes | Serves 4

1 teaspoon extra-virgin olive oil	1 tomato, cored, seeded, and
1 scallion, white and green	diced
parts, finely chopped	2 teaspoons chopped fresh
½ yellow bell pepper, seeded	oregano
and chopped	Sea salt
½ zucchini, diced	Freshly ground black pepper
8 large eggs, beaten	

1. Place a large skillet over medium heat and add the olive oil. 2. Add the scallion, bell pepper, and zucchini to the skillet and sauté for about 5 minutes. 3. Pour in the eggs and, using a wooden spoon or spatula, scramble them until thick, firm curds form and the eggs are cooked through, about 5 minutes. 4. Add the tomato and oregano to the skillet and stir to incorporate. 5. Serve seasoned with salt and pepper.

Per Serving:

calories: 170 | fat: 11g | protein: 14g | carbs: 4g | sugars: 1g | fiber: 1g | sodium: 157mg

Tropical Greek Yogurt Bowl

Prep time: 5 minutes | Cook time: 0 minutes | Serves 2

1½ cups plain low-fat Greek	2 tablespoons halved walnuts
yogurt	1 tablespoon chia seeds
2 kiwis, peeled and sliced	2 teaspoons honey, divided
2 tablespoons shredded	(optional)
unsweetened coconut flakes	

1. Divide the yogurt between two small bowls. 2. Top each serving of yogurt with half of the kiwi slices, coconut flakes, walnuts, chia seeds, and honey (if using).

Per Serving:

calories: 305 | fat: 10g | protein: 14g | carbs: 42g | sugars: 26g | fiber: 7g | sodium: 150mg

Southwestern Egg Casserole

Prep time: 10 minutes | Cook time: 20 minutes | Serves 12

1 cup water	1½ cups shredded 75%-less-fat
2½ cups egg substitute	sharp cheddar cheese
½ cup flour	¼ cup no-trans-fat tub
1 teaspoon baking powder	margarine, melted
⅛ teaspoon salt	2 (4 ounces) cans chopped
⅛ teaspoon pepper	green chilies
2 cups fat-free cottage cheese	

1. Place the steaming rack into the bottom of the inner pot and pour in 1 cup of water. 2. Grease a round springform pan that will fit into the inner pot of the Instant Pot. 3. Combine the egg substitute, flour, baking powder, salt and pepper in a mixing bowl. It will be lumpy. 4. Stir in the cheese, margarine, and green chilies then pour into the springform pan. 5. Place the springform pan onto the steaming rack, close the lid, and secure to the locking position. Be sure the vent is turned to sealing. Set for 20 minutes on Manual at high pressure. 6. Let the pressure release naturally. 7. Carefully remove the springform pan with the handles of the steaming rack and allow to stand 10 minutes before cutting and serving.

Per Serving:

calories: 130 | fat: 4g | protein: 14g | carbs: 9g | sugars: 1g | fiber: 1g | sodium: 450mg

Pumpkin Apple Waffles

Prep time: 10 minutes | Cook time: 20 minutes | Serves 6

2¼ cups whole-wheat pastry	1 teaspoon ground nutmeg
flour	4 eggs
2 tablespoons granulated	1¼ cups pure pumpkin purée
sweetener	1 apple, peeled, cored, and
1 tablespoon baking powder	finely chopped
1 teaspoon ground cinnamon	Melted coconut oil, for cooking

1. In a large bowl, stir together the flour, sweetener, baking powder, cinnamon, and nutmeg. 2. In a small bowl, whisk together the eggs and pumpkin. 3. Add the wet ingredients to the dry and whisk until smooth. 4. Stir the apple into the batter. 5. Cook the waffles according to the waffle maker manufacturer's directions, brushing your waffle iron with melted coconut oil, until all the batter is gone. 6. Serve.

Per Serving:

calories: 241 | fat: 4g | protein: 10g | carbs: 44g | sugars: 7g | fiber: 7g | sodium: 46mg

Creamy Green Smoothie

Prep time: 5 minutes | Cook time: 0 minutes | Serves 2

2 cups shredded kale	milk
½ avocado, diced	¼ cup 2 percent plain Greek
½ Granny Smith apple,	yogurt
unpeeled, cored and chopped	3 ice cubes
1 cup unsweetened almond	

1. Put the kale, avocado, apple, almond milk, yogurt, and ice in a blender and blend until smooth and thick. 2. Pour into two glasses and serve.

Per Serving:

calories: 153 | fat: 9g | protein: 4g | carbs: 15g | sugars: 7g | fiber: 6g | sodium: 117mg

Spanakopita Egg White Frittata

Prep time: 10 minutes | Cook time: 15 minutes | Serves 4

2 tablespoons extra-virgin olive oil
½ sweet onion, chopped
1 red bell pepper, seeded and chopped
½ teaspoon minced garlic
¼ teaspoon sea salt
½ teaspoon freshly ground

black pepper
8 egg whites
2 cups shredded spinach
½ cup crumbled low-sodium feta cheese
1 teaspoon chopped fresh parsley, for garnish

1. Preheat the oven to 375°F. 2. Place a heavy ovenproof skillet over medium-high heat and add the olive oil. 3. Sauté the onion, bell pepper, and garlic until softened, about 5 minutes. Season with salt and pepper. 4. Whisk together the egg whites in a medium bowl, then pour them into the skillet and lightly shake the pan to disburse. 5. Cook the vegetables and eggs for 3 minutes, without stirring. 6. Scatter the spinach over the eggs and sprinkle the feta cheese evenly over the spinach. 7. Put the skillet in the oven and bake, uncovered, until cooked through and firm, about 10 minutes. 8. Loosen the edges of the frittata with a rubber spatula, then invert it onto a plate. 9. Garnish with the chopped parsley and serve.

Per Serving:

calories: 171 | fat: 11g | protein: 11g | carbs: 7g | sugars: 5g | fiber: 1g | sodium: 444mg

Berry–French Toast Stratas

Prep time: 15 minutes | Cook time: 20 to 25 minutes | Serves 6

3 cups assorted fresh berries, such as blueberries, raspberries or cut-up strawberries
1 tablespoon granulated sugar
4 cups cubes (¾ inch) whole wheat bread (about 5 slices)
1½ cups fat-free egg product or 6 eggs

½ cup fat-free (skim) milk
½ cup fat-free half-and-half
2 tablespoons honey
1½ teaspoons vanilla
1 teaspoon ground cinnamon
¼ teaspoon ground nutmeg
½ teaspoon powdered sugar, if desired

1. In medium bowl, mix fruit and granulated sugar; set aside. 2. Heat oven to 350°F. Spray 12 regular-size muffin cups generously with cooking spray. Divide bread cubes evenly among muffin cups. 3. In large bowl, beat remaining ingredients, except powdered sugar, with fork or whisk until well mixed. Pour egg mixture over bread cubes, pushing down lightly with spoon to soak bread cubes. (If all egg mixture doesn't fit into cups, let cups stand up to 10 minutes, gradually adding remaining egg mixture as bread cubes soak it up.) 4. Bake 20 to 25 minutes or until centers are set. Cool 5 minutes. Remove from muffin cups, placing 2 stratas on each of 6 plates. Divide fruit mixture evenly over stratas; sprinkle with powdered sugar.

Per Serving:

calories: 218 | fat: 6g | protein: 11g | carbs: 32g | sugars: 17g | fiber: 4g | sodium: 216mg

Buckwheat Crêpes with Fruit and Yogurt

Prep time: 20 minutes | Cook time: 20 minutes | Serves 5

1½ cups skim milk
3 eggs
1 teaspoon extra-virgin olive oil, plus more for the skillet
1 cup buckwheat flour

½ cup whole-wheat flour
½ cup 2 percent plain Greek yogurt
1 cup sliced strawberries
1 cup blueberries

1. In a large bowl, whisk together the milk, eggs, and 1 teaspoon of oil until well combined. 2. Into a medium bowl, sift together the buckwheat and whole-wheat flours. Add the dry ingredients to the wet ingredients and whisk until well combined and very smooth. 3. Allow the batter to rest for at least 2 hours before cooking. 4. Place a large skillet or crêpe pan over medium-high heat and lightly coat the bottom with oil. 5. Pour about ¼ cup of batter into the skillet. Swirl the pan until the batter completely coats the bottom. 6. Cook the crêpe for about 1 minute, then flip it over. Cook the other side of the crêpe for another minute, until lightly browned. Transfer the cooked crêpe to a plate and cover with a clean dish towel to keep warm. 7. Repeat until the batter is used up; you should have about 10 crêpes. 8. Spoon 1 tablespoon of yogurt onto each crêpe and place two crêpes on each plate. 9. Top with berries and serve.

Per Serving:

calories: 235 | fat: 5g | protein: 12g | carbs: 38g | sugars: 11g | fiber: 5g | sodium: 89mg

White Bean–Oat Waffles

Prep time: 10 minutes | Cook time: 20 minutes | Serves 2

1 large egg white
2 tablespoons finely ground flaxseed
½ cup water
¼ teaspoon salt
1 teaspoon vanilla extract
½ cup cannellini beans, drained

and rinsed
1 teaspoon coconut oil
1 teaspoon liquid stevia
½ cup old-fashioned rolled oats
Extra-virgin olive oil cooking spray

1. In a blender, combine the egg white, flaxseed, water, salt, vanilla, cannellini beans, coconut oil, and stevia. Blend on high for 90 seconds. 2. Add the oats. Blend for 1 minute more. 3. Preheat the waffle iron. The batter will thicken to the correct consistency while the waffle iron preheats. 4. Spray the heated waffle iron with cooking spray. 5. Add ¾ cup of batter. Close the waffle iron. Cook for 6 to 8 minutes, or until done. Repeated with the remaining batter. 6. Serve hot, with your favorite sugar-free topping.

Per Serving:

calories: 294 | fat: 10g | protein: 13g | carbs: 38g | sugars: 4g | fiber: 9g | sodium: 404mg

Gluten-Free Carrot and Oat Pancakes

Prep time: 10 minutes | Cook time: 20 minutes |

Serves 4

1 cup rolled oats
1 cup shredded carrots
1 cup low-fat cottage cheese
2 eggs
½ cup unsweetened plain almond milk
1 teaspoon baking powder

½ teaspoon ground cinnamon
2 tablespoons ground flaxseed
¼ cup plain nonfat Greek yogurt
1 tablespoon pure maple syrup
2 teaspoons canola oil, divided

1. In a blender jar, process the oats until they resemble flour. Add the carrots, cottage cheese, eggs, almond milk, baking powder, cinnamon, and flaxseed to the jar. Process until smooth. 2. In a small bowl, combine the yogurt and maple syrup and stir well. Set aside. 3. In a large skillet, heat 1 teaspoon of oil over medium heat. Using a measuring cup, add ¼ cup of batter per pancake to the skillet. Cook for 1 to 2 minutes until bubbles form on the surface, and flip the pancakes. Cook for another minute until the pancakes are browned and cooked through. Repeat with the remaining 1 teaspoon of oil and remaining batter. 4. Serve warm topped with the maple yogurt.

Per Serving:

calories: 226 | fat: 8g | protein: 15g | carbs: 24g | sugars: 7g | fiber: 4g | sodium: 403mg

Blueberry Cornmeal Muffins

Prep time: 5 minutes | Cook time: 25 minutes |

Makes 12 muffins

2 cups oat flour
½ cup fine corn flour
¼ cup coconut sugar
2 teaspoons baking powder
½ teaspoon baking soda
¼ teaspoon sea salt
1 teaspoon lemon zest
½ cup + 2 to 3 tablespoons

plain nondairy yogurt
¼ cup pure maple syrup
½ cup plain low-fat nondairy milk
1 teaspoon lemon juice or apple cider vinegar
1 cup frozen or fresh blueberries
1 tablespoon oat flour

1. Preheat the oven to 350°F. Line a muffin pan with 12 parchment cupcake liners. 2. In a large bowl, combine the oat flour, corn flour, sugar, baking powder, baking soda, salt, and lemon zest. Stir well. In a medium bowl, combine the yogurt, syrup, milk, and lemon juice or apple cider vinegar, and stir to combine. Add the wet ingredients to the dry and mix until just combined. Toss the berries with the oat flour, and fold them into the batter. Spoon the batter into the muffin liners. Bake for 25 minutes. Remove from the oven and let the muffins cool in the pan for a couple of minutes, then transfer to a cooling rack.

Per Serving:

1 muffin: calorie: 152 | fat: 2g | protein: 4g | carbs: 31g | sugars: 11g | fiber: 3g | sodium: 191mg

Wild Mushroom Frittata

Prep time: 10 minutes | Cook time: 15 minutes |

Serves 4

8 large eggs
½ cup skim milk
¼ teaspoon ground nutmeg
Sea salt
Freshly ground black pepper
2 teaspoons extra-virgin olive oil

2 cups sliced wild mushrooms (cremini, oyster, shiitake, portobello, etc.)
½ red onion, chopped
1 teaspoon minced garlic
½ cup goat cheese, crumbled

1. Preheat the broiler. 2. In a medium bowl, whisk together the eggs, milk, and nutmeg until well combined. Season the egg mixture lightly with salt and pepper and set it aside. 3. Place an ovenproof skillet over medium heat and add the oil, coating the bottom completely by tilting the pan. 4. Sauté the mushrooms, onion, and garlic until translucent, about 7 minutes. 5. Pour the egg mixture into the skillet and cook until the bottom of the frittata is set, lifting the edges of the cooked egg to allow the uncooked egg to seep under. 6. Place the skillet under the broiler until the top is set, about 1 minute. 7. Sprinkle the goat cheese on the frittata and broil until the cheese is melted, about 1 minute more. 8. Remove from the oven. Cut into 4 wedges to serve.

Per Serving:

calories: 258 | fat: 17g | protein: 19g | carbs: 7g | sugars: 3g | fiber: 1g | sodium: 316mg

Oat and Walnut Granola

Prep time: 10 minutes | Cook time: 30 minutes |

Serves 16

4 cups rolled oats
1 cup walnut pieces
½ cup pepitas
¼ teaspoon salt
1 teaspoon ground cinnamon

1 teaspoon ground ginger
½ cup coconut oil, melted
½ cup unsweetened applesauce
1 teaspoon vanilla extract
½ cup dried cherries

1. Preheat the oven to 350°F. Line a baking sheet with parchment paper. 2. In a large bowl, toss the oats, walnuts, pepitas, salt, cinnamon, and ginger. 3. In a large measuring cup, combine the coconut oil, applesauce, and vanilla. Pour over the dry mixture and mix well. 4. Transfer the mixture to the prepared baking sheet. Cook for 30 minutes, stirring about halfway through. Remove from the oven and let the granola sit undisturbed until completely cool. Break the granola into pieces, and stir in the dried cherries. 5. Transfer to an airtight container, and store at room temperature for up to 2 weeks.

Per Serving:

calories: 224| fat: 15g | protein: 5g | carbs: 20g | sugars: 5g | fiber: 3g | sodium: 30mg

Green Nice Cream Breakfast Bowl

Prep time: 5 minutes | Cook time: 0 minutes | Serves 3

3 cups sliced, frozen, overripe banana
1 cup frozen pineapple chunks
2 cups baby spinach
Flesh of 1 ripe avocado (about ½ cup)
Pinch of sea salt

3 to 5 tablespoons low-fat nondairy milk
1 to 2 tablespoons coconut syrup (optional)
½ cup fresh sliced banana
½ cup fresh berries

1. In a blender or food processor, combine the banana, pineapple, spinach, avocado, salt, and 3 tablespoons of the milk. Puree until very smooth. If the mixture is stubborn and not blending, add the additional 2 tablespoons of milk as needed to get the mixture moving. Taste, and add the syrup if desired to sweeten. Spoon the mixture into 3 serving bowls, and top with the banana and berries.

Per Serving:

calorie: 337 | fat: 8g | protein: 5g | carbs: 70g | sugars: 37g | fiber: 12g | sodium: 126mg

Ratatouille Baked Eggs

Prep time: 20 minutes | Cook time: 50 minutes |
Serves 4

2 teaspoons extra-virgin olive oil
½ sweet onion, finely chopped
2 teaspoons minced garlic
½ small eggplant, peeled and diced
1 green zucchini, diced
1 yellow zucchini, diced
1 red bell pepper, seeded and diced

3 tomatoes, seeded and chopped
1 tablespoon chopped fresh oregano
1 tablespoon chopped fresh basil
Pinch red pepper flakes
Sea salt
Freshly ground black pepper
4 large eggs

1. Preheat the oven to 350°F. 2. Place a large ovenproof skillet over medium heat and add the olive oil. 3. Sauté the onion and garlic until softened and translucent, about 3 minutes. Stir in the eggplant and sauté for about 10 minutes, stirring occasionally. Stir in the zucchini and pepper and sauté for 5 minutes. 4. Reduce the heat to low and cover. Cook until the vegetables are soft, about 15 minutes. 5. Stir in the tomatoes, oregano, basil, and red pepper flakes, and cook 10 minutes more. Season the ratatouille with salt and pepper. 6. Use a spoon to create four wells in the mixture. Crack an egg into each well. 7. Place the skillet in the oven and bake until the eggs are firm, about 5 minutes. 8. Remove from the oven. Serve the eggs with a generous scoop of vegetables.

Per Serving:

calories: 164 | fat: 8g | protein: 10g | carbs: 16g | sugars: 8g | fiber: 5g | sodium: 275mg

Broccoli-Mushroom Frittata

Prep time: 10 minutes | Cook time: 20 minutes |
Serves 2

1 tablespoon olive oil
1½ cups broccoli florets, finely chopped
½ cup sliced brown mushrooms
¼ cup finely chopped onion

½ teaspoon salt
¼ teaspoon freshly ground black pepper
6 eggs
¼ cup Parmesan cheese

1. In a nonstick cake pan, combine the olive oil, broccoli, mushrooms, onion, salt, and pepper. Stir until the vegetables are thoroughly coated with oil. Place the cake pan in the air fryer basket and set the air fryer to 400°F (204°C). Air fry for 5 minutes until the vegetables soften. 2. Meanwhile, in a medium bowl, whisk the eggs and Parmesan until thoroughly combined. Pour the egg mixture into the pan and shake gently to distribute the vegetables. Air fry for another 15 minutes until the eggs are set. 3. Remove from the air fryer and let sit for 5 minutes to cool slightly. Use a silicone spatula to gently lift the frittata onto a plate before serving.

Per Serving:

calories: 329 | fat: 23g | protein: 24g | carbs: 6g | fiber: 0g | sodium: 793mg

Cinnamon Wisp Pancakes

Prep time: 5 minutes | Cook time: 10 minutes |
Serves 4

2 cups oat flour
2 tablespoons chia seeds
1 tablespoon baking powder
2 teaspoons cinnamon

Pinch of sea salt
1½ teaspoons vanilla extract
1¾ cups + ¼ cup vanilla low-fat nondairy milk

1. In a large bowl, combine the oat flour, chia seeds, baking powder, cinnamon, and salt. Stir to combine. Add the vanilla and 1¾ cups of the milk, and whisk through the dry mixture until combined. Let the batter sit for a few minutes to thicken. 2. Lightly coat a large nonstick skillet with cooking spray. Heat the pan over medium-high heat for a few minutes until hot, then reduce the heat to medium or medium-low and let it rest for a minute. Using a ladle, scoop ¼ to ⅓ cup of the batter into the pan for each pancake. Depending on the size of pan, cook 2 or 3 pancakes at a time. Cook for several minutes, until small bubbles form on the outer edges and in the centers and the pancakes start to look dry on the top. (Wait until those bubbles form, or the pancakes will be tricky to flip.) Once ready, flip the pancakes to lightly cook the other side for about a minute. Repeat until the batter is all used, adding the extra milk, 1 tablespoon at a time, if needed to thin the batter as you go.

Per Serving:

calorie: 312 | fat: 6g | protein: 11g | carbs: 54g | sugars: 5g | fiber: 9g | sodium: 483mg

Pumpkin Spice Muffins

Prep time: 10 minutes | Cook time: 15 minutes | Serves 6

1 cup blanched finely ground almond flour
½ cup granular erythritol
½ teaspoon baking powder
¼ cup unsalted butter, softened
¼ cup pure pumpkin purée
½ teaspoon ground cinnamon
¼ teaspoon ground nutmeg
1 teaspoon vanilla extract
2 large eggs

1. In a large bowl, mix almond flour, erythritol, baking powder, butter, pumpkin purée, cinnamon, nutmeg, and vanilla. 2. Gently stir in eggs. 3. Evenly pour the batter into six silicone muffin cups. Place muffin cups into the air fryer basket, working in batches if necessary. 4. Adjust the temperature to 300°F (149°C) and bake for 15 minutes. 5. When completely cooked, a toothpick inserted in center will come out mostly clean. Serve warm.

Per Serving:

calories: 261 | fat: 19g | protein: 8g | carbs: 16g | sugars: 11g | fiber: 3g | sodium: 34mg

Pumpkin Walnut Smoothie Bowl

Prep time: 5 minutes | Cook time: 0 minutes | Serves 2

1 cup plain Greek yogurt
½ cup canned pumpkin purée (not pumpkin pie mix)
1 teaspoon pumpkin pie spice
2 (1-gram) packets stevia
½ teaspoon vanilla extract
Pinch sea salt
½ cup chopped walnuts

1. In a bowl, whisk together the yogurt, pumpkin purée, pumpkin pie spice, stevia, vanilla, and salt (or blend in a blender). 2. Spoon into two bowls. Serve topped with the chopped walnuts.

Per Serving:

calories: 277 | fat: 19g | protein: 12g | carbs: 18g | sugars: 11g | fiber: 3g | sodium: 96mg

Bran Apple Muffins

Prep time: 10 minutes | Cook time: 20 minutes | Makes 18 muffins

2 cups whole-wheat flour
1 cup wheat bran
⅓ cup granulated sweetener
1 tablespoon baking powder
2 teaspoons ground cinnamon
½ teaspoon ground ginger
¼ teaspoon ground nutmeg
Pinch sea salt
2 eggs
1½ cups skim milk, at room temperature
½ cup melted coconut oil
2 teaspoons pure vanilla extract
2 apples, peeled, cored, and diced

1. Preheat the oven to 350°F. 2. Line 18 muffin cups with paper liners and set the tray aside. 3. In a large bowl, stir together the flour, bran, sweetener, baking powder, cinnamon, ginger, nutmeg, and salt. 4. In a small bowl, whisk the eggs, milk, coconut oil, and vanilla until blended. 5. Add the wet ingredients to the dry ingredients, stirring until just blended. 6. Stir in the apples and spoon equal amounts of batter into each muffin cup. 7. Bake the muffins until a toothpick inserted in the center of a muffin comes out clean, about 20 minutes. 8. Cool the muffins completely and serve. 9. Store leftover muffins in a sealed container in the refrigerator for up to 3 days or in the freezer for up to 1 month.

Per Serving:

calories: 145 | fat: 7g | protein: 4g | carbs: 19g | sugars: 6g | fiber: 4g | sodium: 17mg

Plum Smoothie

Prep time: 5 minutes | Cook time: 0 minutes | Serves 2

4 ripe plums, pitted
1 cup skim milk
6 ounces 2 percent plain Greek
yogurt
4 ice cubes
¼ teaspoon ground nutmeg

1. Put the plums, milk, yogurt, ice, and nutmeg in a blender and blend until smooth. 2. Pour into two glasses and serve.

Per Serving:

calories: 144 | fat: 1g | protein: 14g | carbs: 20g | sugars: 17g | fiber: 2g | sodium: 82mg

Easy Buckwheat Crêpes

Prep time: 5 minutes | Cook time: 15 minutes | Makes 12 crepes

1 cup buckwheat flour
1¾ cups milk
⅛ teaspoon kosher salt
1 tablespoon extra-virgin olive
oil
½ tablespoon ground flaxseed (optional)

1. Combine the buckwheat flour, milk, salt, extra-virgin olive oil, and flaxseed (if using), in a bowl and whisk thoroughly, or in a blender and pulse until well combined. 2. Heat a nonstick medium skillet over medium heat. Once it's hot, add a ¼ cup of batter to the skillet, spreading it out evenly. Cook until bubbles appear and the edges crisp like a pancake, 1 to 3 minutes, then flip and cook for another 2 minutes. 3. Repeat until all the batter is used up, and the crêpes are cooked. Layer parchment paper or tea towels between the crêpes to keep them from sticking to one another while also keeping them warm until you're ready to eat. 4. Serve with the desired fillings. 5. Store any leftovers in an airtight container in the refrigerator for up to 3 days.

Per Serving:

1 crêpes: calories: 56 | fat: 2g | protein: 2g | carbs: 9g | sugars: 2g | fiber: 1g | sodium: 46mg

Potato-Bacon Gratin

Prep time: 20 minutes | Cook time: 40 minutes |
Serves 8

1 tablespoon olive oil
6 ounces bag fresh spinach
1 clove garlic, minced
4 large potatoes, peeled or unpeeled, divided
6 ounces Canadian bacon slices,

divided
5 ounces reduced-fat grated Swiss cheddar, divided
1 cup lower-sodium, lower-fat chicken broth

1. Set the Instant Pot to Sauté and pour in the olive oil. Cook the spinach and garlic in olive oil just until spinach is wilted (5 minutes or less). Turn off the instant pot. 2. Cut potatoes into thin slices about ¼" thick. 3. In a springform pan that will fit into the inner pot of your Instant Pot, spray it with nonstick spray then layer ⅓ the potatoes, half the bacon, ⅓ the cheese, and half the wilted spinach. 4. Repeat layers ending with potatoes. Reserve ⅓ cheese for later. 5. Pour chicken broth over all. 6. Wipe the bottom of your Instant Pot to soak up any remaining oil, then add in 2 cups of water and the steaming rack. Place the springform pan on top. 7. Close the lid and secure to the locking position. Be sure the vent is turned to sealing. Set for 35 minutes on Manual at high pressure. 8. Perform a quick release. 9. Top with the remaining cheese, then allow to stand 10 minutes before removing from the Instant Pot, cutting and serving.

Per Serving:

calories: 220 | fat: 7g | protein: 14g | carbs: 28g | sugars: 2g | fiber: 3g | sodium: 415mg

Mandarin Orange–Millet Breakfast Bowl

Prep time: 5 minutes | Cook time: 30 minutes |
Serves 2

⅓ cup millet
1 cup nonfat milk
½ cup water
¼ teaspoon cinnamon
¼ teaspoon ground cardamom
1 teaspoon vanilla extract

Pinch salt
Stevia, for sweetening
½ cup canned mandarin oranges, drained
2 tablespoons sliced almonds

1. In a small saucepan set over medium-high heat, stir together the millet, milk, water, cinnamon, cardamom, vanilla, salt, and stevia. Bring to a boil. Reduce the heat to low. Cover and simmer for 25 minutes, without stirring. If the liquid is not completely absorbed, cook for 3 to 5 minutes longer, partially covered. 2. Stir in the oranges. Remove from the heat. 3. Top with the sliced almonds and serve.

Per Serving:

calories: 254 | fat: 7g | protein: 10g | carbs: 38g | sugars: 12g | fiber: 5g | sodium: 73mg

Eggplant Breakfast Sandwich

Prep time: 5 minutes | Cook time: 20 minutes |
Serves 2 to 4

2 tablespoons extra-virgin olive oil, divided
1 eggplant, cut into 8 (½-inch-thick) rounds
¼ teaspoon kosher salt
¼ teaspoon freshly ground

black pepper
4 large eggs
1 garlic clove, minced
4 cups fresh baby spinach
Hot sauce or harissa (optional)

1. Heat 1 tablespoon of extra-virgin olive oil in a large skillet over medium heat. Add the eggplant in a single layer and cook until tender and browned on both sides, 4 to 5 minutes per side. Transfer the eggplant from the skillet to a plate and season it with salt and pepper. Wipe out the skillet and set aside. 2. Meanwhile, place a large saucepan filled three-quarters full with water over medium-high heat and bring it to a simmer. Carefully break the eggs into small, individual bowls and pour slowly into a fine-mesh strainer over another bowl. Allow the excess white to drain, then lower the strainer into the water. Tilt the egg out into the water. Repeat with the remaining eggs. Swirl the water occasionally as the eggs cook and whites set, about 4 minutes. Remove the eggs with a slotted spoon, transfer them to a paper towel, and drain. 3. Heat the remaining 1 tablespoon of extra-virgin olive oil over medium heat in the large skillet and add the garlic and spinach. Cook until the spinach is wilted, about 1 minute. 4. Place one eggplant round on each of four plates and evenly divide the spinach among the rounds. Top the spinach with a poached egg on each sandwich and place the remaining eggplant round on the egg. Serve with hot sauce or harissa (if using).

Per Serving:

calories: 174 | fat: 12g | protein: 9g | carbs: 10g | sugars: 5g | fiber: 5g | sodium: 243mg

Instant Pot Hard-Boiled Eggs

Prep time: 10 minutes | Cook time: 5 minutes |
Serves 7

1 cup water   6 to 8 eggs

1. Pour the water into the inner pot. Place the eggs in a steamer basket or rack that came with pot. 2. Close the lid and secure to the locking position. Be sure the vent is turned to sealing. Set for 5 minutes on Manual at high pressure. (It takes about 5 minutes for pressure to build and then 5 minutes to cook.) 3. Let pressure naturally release for 5 minutes, then do quick pressure release. 4. Place hot eggs into cool water to halt cooking process. You can peel cooled eggs immediately or refrigerate unpeeled.

Per Serving:

calories: 72 | fat: 5g | protein: 6g | carbs: 0g | sugars: 0g | fiber: 0g | sodium: 71mg

Easy Breakfast Chia Pudding

Prep time: 5 minutes | Cook time: 0 minutes | Serves 4

4 cups unsweetened almond milk or skim milk
¾ cup chia seeds

1 teaspoon ground cinnamon
Pinch sea salt

1. Stir together the milk, chia seeds, cinnamon, and salt in a medium bowl. 2. Cover the bowl with plastic wrap and chill in the refrigerator until the pudding is thick, about 1 hour. 3. Sweeten with your favorite sweetener and fruit.

Per Serving:

calories: 129 | fat: 3g | protein: 10g | carbs: 16g | sugars: 12g | fiber: 3g | sodium: 131mg

Avocado Toast With Tomato And Cottage Cheese

Prep time: 5 minutes | Cook time: 0 minutes | Serves 2

½ cup cottage cheese
½ avocado, mashed
1 teaspoon Dijon mustard
Dash hot sauce (optional)

2 slices whole-grain bread, toasted
2 slices tomato

1. In a small bowl, mix together the cottage cheese, avocado, mustard, and hot sauce, if using, until well mixed. 2. Spread the mixture on the toast. 3. Top each piece of toast with a tomato slice.

Per Serving:

calories: 195 | fat: 9g | protein: 12g | carbs: 18g | sugars: 4g | fiber: 6g | sodium: 362mg

Western Omelet

Prep time: 5 minutes | Cook time: 10 minutes | Serves 2

1½ teaspoons canola oil
¾ cup egg whites
¼ cup minced lean ham
2 tablespoons minced green bell

pepper
2 tablespoons minced onion
⅛ teaspoon freshly ground black pepper

1. In a medium nonstick skillet over medium-low heat, heat the oil. 2. In a small mixing bowl, beat the egg whites slightly, and add the remaining ingredients along with a dash of salt, if desired. Pour the egg mixture into the heated skillet. 3. When the omelet begins to set, gently lift the edges of the omelet with a spatula, and tilt the skillet to allow the uncooked portion to flow underneath. Continue cooking until the eggs are firm. Then transfer to a serving platter.

Per Serving:

calories: 107 | fat: 4g | protein: 14g | carbs: 2g | sugars: 1g | fiber: 0g | sodium: 367mg

Golden Potato Cakes

Prep time: 10 minutes | Cook time: 25 minutes | Serves 4

½ pound russet potatoes, peeled, shredded, rinsed, and patted dry
¼ sweet onion, chopped
1 teaspoon extra-virgin olive oil

1 teaspoon chopped fresh thyme
Sea salt
Freshly ground black pepper
Nonstick cooking spray
1 cup unsweetened applesauce

1. Place the potatoes, onion, oil, and thyme in a large bowl and stir to mix well. 2. Season the potato mixture generously with salt and pepper. 3. Place a large skillet over medium heat and lightly coat it with cooking spray. 4. Scoop about ¼ cup of potato mixture per cake into the skillet and press down with a spatula, about 4 cakes per batch. 5. Cook until the bottoms are golden brown and firm, about 5 to 7 minutes, then flip the cake over. Cook the other side until it is golden brown and the cake is completely cooked through, about 5 minutes more. 6. Remove the cakes to a plate and repeat with the remaining mixture. 7. Serve with the applesauce.

Per Serving:

calories: 88 | fat: 1g | protein: 1g | carbs: 19g | sugars: 7g | fiber: 2g | sodium: 6mg

Cinnamon French Toast

Prep time: 10 minutes | Cook time: 20 minutes | Serves 8

3 eggs
2 cups low-fat milk
2 tablespoons maple syrup
15 drops liquid stevia
2 teaspoons vanilla extract
2 teaspoons cinnamon

Pinch salt
16 ounces whole wheat bread, cubed and left out overnight to go stale
1½ cups water

1. In a medium bowl, whisk together the eggs, milk, maple syrup, Stevia, vanilla, cinnamon, and salt. Stir in the cubes of whole wheat bread. 2. You will need a 7-inch round baking pan for this. Spray the inside with nonstick spray, then pour the bread mixture into the pan. 3. Place the trivet in the bottom of the inner pot, then pour in the water. 4. Make foil sling and insert it onto the trivet. Carefully place the 7-inch pan on top of the foil sling/trivet. 5. Secure the lid to the locked position, then make sure the vent is turned to sealing. 6. Press the Manual button and use the "+/-" button to set the Instant Pot for 20 minutes. 7. When cook time is up, let the Instant Pot release naturally for 5 minutes, then quick release the rest

Per Serving:

calories: 75 | fat: 3g | protein: 4g | carbs: 7g | sugars: 6g | fiber: 0g | sodium: 74mg

Cheesy Scrambled Eggs

Prep time: 2 minutes | Cook time: 9 minutes | Serves 2

1 teaspoon unsalted butter
2 large eggs
2 tablespoons milk
2 tablespoons shredded Cheddar

cheese
Salt and freshly ground black
pepper, to taste

1. Preheat the air fryer to 300°F (149°C). Place the butter in a baking pan and cook for 1 to 2 minutes, until melted. 2. In a small bowl, whisk together the eggs, milk, and cheese. Season with salt and black pepper. Transfer the mixture to the pan. 3. Cook for 3 minutes. Stir the eggs and push them toward the center of the pan. 4. Cook for another 2 minutes, then stir again. Cook for another 2 minutes, until the eggs are just cooked. Serve warm.

Per Serving:

calories: 122 | fat: 9g | protein: 9g | carbs: 1g | sugars: 1g | fiber: 0g | sodium: 357mg

Cranberry Almond Grits

Prep time: 10 minutes | Cook time: 10 minutes |

Serves 5

¾ cup stone-ground grits or
polenta (not instant)
½ cup unsweetened dried
cranberries
Pinch kosher salt

1 tablespoon unsalted butter or
ghee (optional)
1 tablespoon half-and-half
¼ cup sliced almonds, toasted

1. In the electric pressure cooker, stir together the grits, cranberries, salt, and 3 cups of water. 2. Close and lock the lid. Set the valve to sealing. 3. Cook on high pressure for 10 minutes. 4. When the cooking is complete, hit Cancel and quick release the pressure. 5. Once the pin drops, unlock and remove the lid. 6. Add the butter (if using) and half-and-half. Stir until the mixture is creamy, adding more half-and-half if necessary. 7. Spoon into serving bowls and sprinkle with almonds.

Per Serving:

calories: 218 | fat: 10g | protein: 5g | carbs: 32g | sugars: 7g | fiber: 4g | sodium: 28mg

Oatmeal Strawberry Smoothie

Prep time: 5 minutes | Cook time: 0 minutes | Serves 2

2 tablespoons instant oats
1 cup frozen strawberries

3 cups skim milk
½ teaspoon pure vanilla extract

1. Put the oats, strawberries, milk, and vanilla in a blender and blend until smooth. 2. Pour into two glasses and serve.

Per Serving:

calories: 179 | fat: 1g | protein: 14g | carbs: 27g | sugars: 18g | fiber: 3g | sodium: 156mg

Cynthia's Yogurt

Prep time: 10 minutes | Cook time: 8 hours | Serves 16

1 gallon low-fat milk
¼ cup low-fat plain yogurt with active cultures

1. Pour milk into the inner pot of the Instant Pot. 2. Lock lid, move vent to sealing, and press the yogurt button. Press Adjust till it reads "boil." 3. When boil cycle is complete (about 1 hour), check the temperature. It should be at 185°F. If it's not, use the Sauté function to warm to 185. 4. After it reaches 185°F, unplug Instant Pot, remove inner pot, and cool. You can place on cooling rack and let it slowly cool. If in a hurry, submerge the base of the pot in cool water. Cool milk to 110°F. 5. When mixture reaches 110, stir in the ¼ cup of yogurt. Lock the lid in place and move vent to sealing. 6. Press Yogurt. Use the Adjust button until the screen says 8:00. This will now incubate for 8 hours. 7. After 8 hours (when the cycle is finished), chill yogurt, or go immediately to straining in step 8. 8. After chilling, or following the 8 hours, strain the yogurt using a nut milk bag. This will give it the consistency of Greek yogurt.

Per Serving:

calories: 141 | fat: 5g | protein: 10g | carbs: 14g | sugars: 1g | fiber: 0g | sodium: 145mg

Veggie And Egg White Scramble With Pepper Jack Cheese

Prep time: 5 minutes | Cook time: 10 minutes |

Serves 2

2 tablespoons extra-virgin olive
oil
½ red onion, finely chopped
1 green bell pepper, seeded and
finely chopped
8 large egg whites (or 4 whole

large eggs), beaten
½ teaspoon sea salt
2 ounces grated pepper Jack
cheese
Salsa (optional, for serving)

1. In a medium nonstick skillet over medium-high heat, heat the olive oil until it shimmers. 2. Add the onion and bell pepper and cook, stirring occasionally, until the vegetables begin to brown, about 5 minutes. 3. Meanwhile, in a small bowl, whisk together the egg whites and salt. 4. Add the egg whites to the pan and cook, stirring, until the whites set, about 3 minutes. Add the cheese. Cook, stirring, 1 minute more. 5. Serve topped with salsa, if desired.

Per Serving:

calories: 320 | fat: 23g | protein: 22g | carbs: 7g | sugars: 4g | fiber: 2g | sodium: 584mg

Chapter 3 Beans and Grains

Curried Rice with Pineapple

Prep time: 5 minutes | Cook time: 35 minutes |

Serves 8

1 onion, chopped
1½ cups water
1¼ cups low-sodium chicken broth
1 cup uncooked brown basmati rice, soaked in water 20 minutes and drained before cooking
2 red bell peppers, minced

1 teaspoon curry powder
1 teaspoon ground turmeric
1 teaspoon ground ginger
2 garlic cloves, minced
One 8 ounces can pineapple chunks packed in juice, drained
¼ cup sliced almonds, toasted

1. In a medium saucepan, combine the onion, water, and chicken broth. Bring to a boil, and add the rice, peppers, curry powder, turmeric, ginger, and garlic. Cover, placing a paper towel in between the pot and the lid, and reduce the heat. Simmer for 25 minutes. 2. Add the pineapple, and continue to simmer 5 to 7 minutes more until rice is tender and water is absorbed. Taste and add salt, if desired. Transfer to a serving bowl, and garnish with almonds to serve.

Per Serving:

calorie: 144 | fat: 3g | protein: 4g | carbs: 27g | sugars: 6g | fiber: 3g | sodium: 16mg

Colorful Rice Casserole

Prep time: 5 minutes | Cook time: 20 minutes |

Serves 12

1 tablespoon extra-virgin olive oil
1½ pounds zucchini, thinly sliced
¾ cup chopped scallions
2 cups corn kernels (frozen or fresh; if frozen, defrost)
One 14½ ounces can no-salt-

added chopped tomatoes, undrained
¼ cup chopped parsley
1 teaspoon oregano
3 cups cooked brown (or white) rice
⅛ teaspoon freshly ground black pepper

1. In a large skillet, heat the oil. Add the zucchini and scallions, and sauté for 5 minutes. 2. Add the remaining ingredients, cover, reduce heat, and simmer for 10 to 15 minutes or until the vegetables are heated through. Season with salt, if desired, and pepper. Transfer to a bowl, and serve.

Per Serving:

calorie: 109 | fat: 2g | protein: 3g | carbs: 21g | sugars: 4g | fiber: 3g | sodium: 14mg

BBQ Lentils

Prep time: 10 minutes | Cook time: 55 minutes |

Serves 5

2 cups dried green or brown lentils, rinsed
3 tablespoons balsamic vinegar
4½ cups water
½ cup tomato paste
2 tablespoons vegan Worcestershire sauce

2 teaspoons dried rosemary
1 teaspoon onion powder
½ teaspoon garlic powder
½ teaspoon allspice
¼ teaspoon sea salt
1 tablespoon coconut nectar or pure maple syrup

1. In a large saucepan over medium-high heat, combine the lentils with 2 tablespoons of the vinegar. Cook, stirring, for 5 to 7 minutes to lightly toast the lentils. Once the pan is getting dry, add the water, tomato paste, Worcestershire sauce, rosemary, onion powder, garlic powder, allspice, salt, nectar or syrup, and the remaining 1 tablespoon vinegar, and stir through. Bring to a boil, then reduce the heat to low, cover the pot, and cook for 37 to 40 minutes, or until the lentils are fully tender. Season to taste, and serve.

Per Serving:

calorie: 295 | fat: 1g | protein: 20g | carbs: 54g | sugars: 9g | fiber: 14g | sodium: 399mg

Beet Greens and Black Beans

Prep time: 10 minutes | Cook time: 20 minutes |

Serves 4

1 tablespoon unsalted non-hydrogenated plant-based butter
½ Vidalia onion, thinly sliced
½ cup store-bought low-sodium vegetable broth
1 bunch beet greens, cut into

ribbons
1 bunch dandelion greens, cut into ribbons
1 (15 ounces) can no-salt-added black beans
Freshly ground black pepper

1. In a medium skillet, melt the butter over low heat. 2. Add the onion, and sauté for 3 to 5 minutes, or until the onion is translucent. 3. Add the broth and greens. Cover the skillet and cook for 7 to 10 minutes, or until the greens are wilted. 4. Add the black beans and cook for 3 to 5 minutes, or until the beans are tender. Season with black pepper.

Per Serving:

calorie: 153 | fat: 3g | protein: 9g | carbs: 25g | sugars: 2g | fiber: 11g | sodium: 312mg

Chicken–Wild Rice Salad with Dried Cherries

Prep time: 30 minutes | Cook time: 10 minutes |
Serves 5

1 package (6.2 ounces) fast-cooking long-grain and wild rice mix
2 cups chopped cooked chicken or turkey
1 medium unpeeled apple, chopped (1 cup)
1 medium green bell pepper, chopped (1 cup)
1 medium stalk celery, chopped

(½ cup)
½ cup chopped dried apricots
⅓ cup chopped dried cherries
2 tablespoons reduced-sodium soy sauce
2 tablespoons water
2 teaspoons sugar
2 teaspoons cider vinegar
⅓ cup dry-roasted peanuts

1. Cook rice mix as directed on package, omitting butter. On large cookie sheet, spread rice evenly in thin layer. Let stand 10 minutes, stirring occasionally, until cool. 2. Meanwhile, in large bowl, mix chicken, apple, bell pepper, celery, apricots and cherries. In small bowl, mix soy sauce, water, sugar and vinegar until sugar is dissolved. 3. Add rice and soy sauce mixture to apple mixture; toss gently until coated. Add peanuts; toss gently.

Per Serving:
calorie: 380 | fat: 7g | protein: 24g | carbs: 54g | sugars: 21g | fiber: 4g | sodium: 760mg

Veggies and Kasha with Balsamic Vinaigrette

Prep time: 15 minutes | Cook time: 8 minutes |
Serves 4

Salad
1 cup water
½ cup uncooked buckwheat kernels or groats (kasha)
4 medium green onions, thinly sliced (¼ cup)
Vinaigrette
2 tablespoons balsamic or red wine vinegar
1 tablespoon olive oil
2 teaspoons sugar

2 medium tomatoes, seeded, coarsely chopped (1½ cups)
1 medium unpeeled cucumber, seeded, chopped (1¼ cups)

½ teaspoon salt
¼ teaspoon pepper
1 clove garlic, finely chopped

1. In 8-inch skillet, heat water to boiling. Add kasha; cook over medium-high heat 7 to 8 minutes, stirring occasionally, until tender. Drain if necessary. 2. In large bowl, mix kasha and remaining salad ingredients. 3. In tightly covered container, shake vinaigrette ingredients until blended. Pour vinaigrette over kasha mixture; toss. Cover; refrigerate 1 to 2 hours to blend flavors.

Per Serving:
calorie: 120 | fat: 4g | protein: 2g | carbs: 19g | sugars: 6g | fiber: 3g | sodium: 310mg

Veggie Unfried Rice

Prep time: 15 minutes | Cook time: 25 minutes |
Serves 4

1 tablespoon extra-virgin olive oil
1 bunch collard greens, stemmed and cut into chiffonade
½ cup store-bought low-sodium vegetable broth
1 carrot, cut into 2-inch

matchsticks
1 red onion, thinly sliced
1 garlic clove, minced
2 tablespoons coconut aminos
1 cup cooked brown rice
1 large egg
1 teaspoon red pepper flakes
1 teaspoon paprika

1. In a large Dutch oven, heat the olive oil over medium heat. 2. Add the collard greens and cook for 3 to 5 minutes, or until the greens are wilted. 3. Add the broth, carrot, onion, garlic, and coconut aminos, then cover and cook for 5 to 7 minutes, or until the carrot softens and the onion and garlic are translucent. 4. Uncover, add the rice, and cook for 3 to 5 minutes, gently mixing all the ingredients together until well combined but not mushy. 5. Crack the egg over the pot and gently scramble the egg. Cook for 2 to 5 minutes, or until the eggs are no longer runny. 6. Remove from the heat and season with the red pepper flakes and paprika.

Per Serving:
calorie: 164 | fat: 4g | protein: 9g | carbs: 26g | sugars: 3g | fiber: 9g | sodium: 168mg

Green Chickpea Falafel

Prep time: 10 minutes | Cook time: 11 to 12 minutes | Serves 4

1 bag (14 ounces) green chickpeas, thawed (about 3½ cups)
½ cup fresh flat-leaf parsley leaves
½ cup fresh cilantro leaves
1½ tablespoons freshly squeezed lemon juice

2 medium-large cloves garlic
2 teaspoons ground cumin
½ teaspoon turmeric
1 teaspoon ground coriander
1 teaspoon sea salt
¼ to ½ teaspoon crushed red-pepper flakes
1 cup rolled oats

1. In a food processor, combine the chickpeas, parsley, cilantro, lemon juice, garlic, cumin, turmeric, coriander, salt, and red-pepper flakes. (Use ¼ teaspoon if you like it mild and ½ teaspoon if you like it spicier.) Process until the mixture breaks down and begins to smooth out. Add the oats and pulse a few times to work them in. Refrigerate for 30 minutes, if possible. 2. Preheat the oven to 400°F. Line a baking sheet with parchment paper. 3. Use a cookie scoop to take small scoops of the mixture, 1 to 1½ tablespoons each. Place falafel balls on the prepared baking sheet. Bake for 11 to 12 minutes, until the falafel balls begin to firm (they will still be tender inside) and turn golden in spots.

Per Serving:
calorie: 253 | fat: 4g | protein: 12g | carbs: 43g | sugars: 5g | fiber: 10g | sodium: 601mg

Rice with Spinach and Feta

Prep time: 10 minutes | Cook time: 15 minutes |

Serves 4

¾ cup uncooked brown rice
1½ cups water
1 tablespoon extra-virgin olive oil
1 medium onion, diced
1 cup sliced mushrooms
2 garlic cloves, minced
1 tablespoon lemon juice

½ teaspoon dried oregano
9 cups fresh spinach, stems trimmed, washed, patted dry, and coarsely chopped
⅓ cup crumbled fat-free feta cheese
⅛ teaspoon freshly ground black pepper

1. In a medium saucepan over medium heat, combine the rice and water. Bring to a boil, cover, reduce heat, and simmer for 15 minutes. Transfer to a serving bowl. 2. In a skillet, heat the oil. Sauté the onion, mushrooms, and garlic for 5 to 7 minutes. Stir in the lemon juice and oregano. Add the spinach, cheese, and pepper, tossing until the spinach is slightly wilted. 3. Toss with rice and serve.

Per Serving:

calorie: 205 | fat: 5g | protein: 7g | carbs: 34g | sugars: 2g | fiber: 4g | sodium: 129mg

Baked Vegetable Macaroni Pie

Prep time: 15 minutes | Cook time: 35 minutes |

Serves 6

1 (16 ounces) package whole-wheat macaroni
1 small yellow onion, chopped
2 garlic cloves, minced
2 celery stalks, thinly sliced
¼ teaspoon freshly ground black pepper
2 tablespoons chickpea flour

1 cup fat-free milk
2 cups grated reduced-fat sharp Cheddar cheese
2 large zucchini, finely grated and squeezed dry
2 roasted red peppers, chopped into ¼-inch pieces

1. Preheat the oven to 350°F. 2. Bring a large pot of water to a boil. 3. Add the macaroni and cook for 2 to 5 minutes, or until al dente. 4. Drain the macaroni, reserving 1 cup of the pasta water for the cheese sauce. Rinse under cold running water, and transfer to a large bowl. 5. In a large cast iron skillet, warm the pasta water over medium heat. 6. Add the onion, garlic, celery, and pepper. Cook for 3 to 5 minutes, or until the onion is translucent. 7. Add the chickpea flour slowly, mixing often. 8. Stir in the milk and cheese until a thick liquid is formed. It should be about the consistency of a smoothie. 9. Add the pasta to the cheese mixture along with the zucchini and red peppers. Mix thoroughly so the ingredients are evenly dispersed. 10. Cover the skillet tightly with aluminum foil, transfer to the oven, and bake for 15 to 20 minutes, or until the cheese is well melted. 11. Uncover and bake for 5 minutes, or until golden brown.

Per Serving:

calorie: 382 | fat: 4g | protein: 24g | carbs: 67g | sugars: 6g | fiber: 8g | sodium: 373mg

Southwestern Quinoa Salad

Prep time: 15 minutes | Cook time: 25 minutes |

Serves 6

Salad
1 cup uncooked quinoa
1 large onion, chopped (1 cup)
1½ cups reduced-sodium chicken broth
1 cup packed fresh cilantro leaves
¼ cup raw unsalted hulled pumpkin seeds (pepitas)
2 cloves garlic, sliced
Garnish
1 avocado, pitted, peeled, thinly sliced

⅛ teaspoon ground cumin
2 tablespoons chopped green chiles (from 4.5-oz can)
1 tablespoon olive oil
1 can (15 ounces) no-salt-added black beans, drained, rinsed
6 medium plum (Roma) tomatoes, chopped (2 cups)
2 tablespoons lime juice

4 small cilantro sprigs

1 Rinse quinoa thoroughly by placing in a fine-mesh strainer and holding under cold running water until water runs clear; drain well. 2 Spray 3-quart saucepan with cooking spray. Heat over medium heat. Add onion to pan; cook 6 to 8 minutes, stirring occasionally, until golden brown. Stir in quinoa and chicken broth. Heat to boiling; reduce heat. Cover and simmer 10 to 15 minutes or until all liquid is absorbed; remove from heat. 3 Meanwhile, in small food processor*, place cilantro, pumpkin seeds, garlic and cumin. Cover; process 5 to 10 seconds, using quick on-and-off motions; scrape side. Add chiles and oil. Cover; process, using quick on-and-off motions, until paste forms. 4 To cooked quinoa, add pesto mixture and the remaining salad ingredients. Refrigerate at least 30 minutes to blend flavors. 5 To serve, divide salad evenly among 4 plates; top each serving with 3 or 4 slices avocado and 1 sprig cilantro.

Per Serving:

calorie: 310 | fat: 12g | protein: 13g | carbs: 38g | sugars: 5g | fiber: 9g | sodium: 170mg

Asian Fried Rice

Prep time: 5 minutes | Cook time: 20 minutes |

Serves 4

2 tablespoons peanut oil
¼ cup chopped onion
1 cup sliced carrot
1 green bell pepper, diced
1 tablespoon grated fresh ginger
2 cups cooked brown rice, cold

½ cup water chestnuts, drained
½ cup sliced mushrooms
1 tablespoon light soy sauce
2 egg whites
½ cup sliced scallions

1. In a large skillet, heat the oil. Sauté the onion, carrot, green pepper, and ginger for 5 to 6 minutes. 2. Stir in the rice, water chestnuts, mushrooms, and soy sauce, and stir-fry for 8 to 10 minutes. 3. Stir in the egg whites, and continue to stir-fry for another 3 minutes. Top with the sliced scallions to serve.

Per Serving:

calorie: 223 | fat: 9g | protein: 6g | carbs: 32g | sugars: 5g | fiber: 4g | sodium: 151mg

BBQ Bean Burgers

Prep time: 10 minutes | Cook time: 20 minutes |
Makes 8 burgers

2 cups sliced carrots
1 medium-large clove garlic, quartered
1 can (15 ounces) kidney beans, rinsed and drained
1 cup cooked, cooled brown rice
¼ cup barbecue sauce
½ tablespoon vegan

Worcestershire sauce
½ tablespoon Dijon mustard
Scant ½ teaspoon sea salt
¼ to ½ teaspoon smoked paprika
1 tablespoon chopped fresh thyme
1¼ cups rolled oats

1. In a food processor, combine the carrots and garlic. Pulse until minced. Add the beans, rice, barbecue sauce, Worcestershire sauce, mustard, salt, paprika, and thyme. Puree until well combined. Once the mixture is fairly smooth, add the oats and pulse to combine. Chill the mixture for 30 minutes, if possible. 2. Preheat the oven to 400°F. Line a baking sheet with parchment paper. 3. Use an ice cream scoop to scoop the mixture onto the prepared baking sheet, flattening to shape it into patties. Bake for about 20 minutes, flipping the burgers halfway through. Alternatively, you can cook the burgers in a nonstick skillet over medium heat for 6 to 8 minutes Per side, or until golden brown.

Per Serving:

calorie: 152 | fat: 2g | protein: 6g | carbs: 29g | sugars: 6 | fiber: 5g | sodium: 247mg

Chicken and Vegetables with Quinoa

Prep time: 25 minutes | Cook time: 25 minutes |
Serves 4

1⅓ cups uncooked quinoa
2⅔ cups water
⅔ cup chicken broth
2 cups 1-inch pieces fresh green beans
½ cup ready-to-eat baby-cut carrots, cut in half lengthwise
1 tablespoon olive oil
½ lb boneless skinless chicken

breasts, cut into bite-size pieces
½ cup bite-size strips red bell pepper
½ cup sliced fresh mushrooms
½ teaspoon dried rosemary leaves
¼ teaspoon salt
2 cloves garlic, finely chopped

1 Rinse quinoa thoroughly by placing in a fine-mesh strainer and holding under cold running water until water runs clear; drain well. 2 In 2-quart saucepan, heat water to boiling. Add quinoa; return to boiling. Reduce heat to low. Cover; cook 12 to 16 minutes or until liquid is absorbed. 3 Meanwhile, in 12-inch nonstick skillet, heat broth to boiling over high heat. Add green beans and carrots. Reduce heat to medium-high. Cover; cook 5 to 7 minutes or until vegetables are crisp-tender. 4 Stir oil, chicken, bell pepper, mushrooms, rosemary, salt and garlic into vegetables. Cook over medium-high heat 8 to 9 minutes, stirring frequently, until chicken is no longer pink in center. Serve over quinoa.

Per Serving:

calorie: 350 | fat: 9g | protein: 22g | carbs: 46g | sugars: 6g | fiber: 6g | sodium: 380mg

Spicy Couscous and Chickpea Salad

Prep time: 20 minutes | Cook time: 10 minutes |
Serves 4

Salad
½ cup uncooked whole wheat couscous
1½ cups water
¼ teaspoon salt
1 can (15 ounces) chickpeas (garbanzo beans), drained, rinsed
1 can (14½ ounces) diced tomatoes with green chiles, undrained
½ cup frozen shelled edamame

(green soybeans) or lima beans, thawed
2 tablespoons chopped fresh cilantro
Green bell peppers, halved, if desired
Dressing
2 tablespoons olive oil
1 teaspoon ground coriander
½ teaspoon ground cumin
½ teaspoon ground cinnamon

1. Cook couscous in the water and salt as directed on package. 2. Meanwhile, in medium bowl, mix chickpeas, tomatoes, edamame and cilantro. In small bowl, mix dressing ingredients until well blended. 3. Add cooked couscous to salad; mix well. Pour dressing over salad; stir gently to mix. Spoon salad mixture into halved bell peppers. Serve immediately, or cover and refrigerate until serving time.

Per Serving:

calorie: 370 | fat: 11g | protein: 16g | carbs: 53g | sugars: 6g | fiber: 10g | sodium: 460mg

Pressure-Stewed Chickpeas

Prep time: 10 minutes | Cook time: 25 minutes |
Serves 5

3 tablespoons water
2 large or 3 small to medium onions, chopped (3 to 3½ cups)
1½ tablespoons smoked paprika
½ teaspoon ground cumin
⅛ to ¼ teaspoon ground allspice

Rounded ½ teaspoon sea salt
2 cans (15 ounces each) chickpeas, rinsed and drained
⅔ cup chopped, pitted dates
1 jar (24 ounces) strained tomatoes

1. In the instant pot set on the sauté function, combine the water, onions, paprika, cumin, allspice, and salt. Cook for 6 to 7 minutes, stirring occasionally. If the mixture is sticking, add another tablespoon or two of water. Add the chickpeas, dates, and tomatoes, and stir well. Turn off the sauté function, and put on the lid. Manually set to pressure cook on high for 18 minutes. Release the pressure or let the pressure release naturally. Stir, taste, season as desired, and serve.

Per Serving:

calorie: 258 | fat: 4g | protein: 10g | carbs: 50g | sugars: 23g | fiber: 13g | sodium: 742mg

Brown Rice–Stuffed Butternut Squash

Prep time: 30 minutes | Cook time: 50 minutes |
Serves 4

2 small butternut squash (about 2 lb each)	1 thyme sprig
4 teaspoons olive oil	1 bay leaf
¼ teaspoon salt	2 links (3 ounces each) sweet
½ teaspoon freshly ground pepper	Italian turkey sausage, casings removed
⅓ cup uncooked brown basmati rice	1 small onion, chopped (⅓ cup)
1¼ cups reduced-sodium chicken broth	1 cup sliced cremini mushrooms
	1 cup fresh baby spinach leaves
	1 teaspoon chopped fresh or ¼ teaspoon dried sage leaves

1 Heat oven to 375°F. Cut each squash lengthwise in half; remove seeds and fibers. Drizzle cut sides with 3 teaspoons of the olive oil; sprinkle with salt and pepper. On cookie sheet, place squash, cut side down. Bake 35 to 40 minutes, until squash is tender at thickest portion when pierced with fork. When cool enough to handle, cut off long ends of squash to within ½ inch edge of cavities (peel and refrigerate ends for another use). 2 Meanwhile, in 1-quart saucepan, heat remaining 1 teaspoon oil over medium heat. Add rice to oil, stirring well to coat. Stir in chicken broth, thyme and bay leaf. Heat to boiling; reduce heat. Cover and simmer 30 to 35 minutes, until all liquid is absorbed and rice is tender. Remove from heat; discard thyme sprig and bay leaf. 3 In 10-inch nonstick skillet, cook sausage and onion over medium-high heat 8 to 10 minutes, stirring frequently, until sausage is thoroughly cooked. Add mushrooms. Cook 4 minutes or until mushrooms are tender. Stir in cooked rice, spinach and sage; cook about 3 minutes or until spinach is wilted and mixture is hot. Divide sausage-rice mixture between squash halves, pressing down on filling so it forms a slight mound over cavity.

Per Serving:

calorie: 350 | fat: 10g | protein: 14g | carbs: 50g | sugars: 14g | fiber: 5g | sodium: 670mg

Farmers' Market Barley Risotto

Prep time: 30 minutes | Cook time: 15 minutes |
Serves 4

1 tablespoon olive oil	chicken broth
1 medium onion, chopped (½ cup)	2 cups reduced-sodium chicken broth
1 medium bell pepper, coarsely chopped (1 cup)	3 cups water
2 cups chopped fresh mushrooms (4 ounces)	1½ cups grape tomatoes, cut in half (if large, cut into quarters)
1 cup frozen whole-kernel corn	⅔ cup shredded Parmesan cheese
1 cup uncooked medium pearled barley	3 tablespoons chopped fresh or 1 teaspoon dried basil leaves
¼ cup dry white wine or	½ teaspoon pepper

1 In 4-quart Dutch oven or saucepan, heat oil over medium heat. Cook onion, bell pepper, mushrooms and corn in oil about 5 minutes, stirring frequently, until onion is crisp-tender. Add barley, stirring about 1 minute to coat. 2 Stir in wine and ½ cup of the broth. Cook 5 minutes, stirring frequently, until liquid is almost absorbed. Repeat with remaining broth and 3 cups water, adding ½ to ¾ cup of broth or water at a time and stirring frequently, until absorbed. 3 Stir in tomatoes, ¼ cup of the cheese, the basil and pepper. Cook until thoroughly heated. Sprinkle with remaining ¼ cup cheese.

Per Serving:

calorie: 370 | fat: 8g | protein: 15g | carbs: 55g | sugars: 6g | fiber: 11g | sodium: 520mg

Dirty Forbidden Rice

Prep time: 15 minutes | Cook time: 35 minutes |
Serves 10

1 pound 90 percent lean ground beef	2 large carrots, peeled and chopped
1 small red onion, chopped	2⅔ cups (15 ounces) forbidden rice (black rice)
1 medium tomato, chopped	4¾ cups store-bought low-sodium chicken broth
1 garlic clove, minced	1 tablespoon Creole seasoning
½ large red bell pepper, chopped	

1. Heat a Dutch oven over medium heat. 2. Put the ground beef, onion, tomato, and garlic in the pot and cook for 5 minutes, or until the beef is browned. 3. Stir in the bell pepper, carrots, and rice. 4. Add the broth and Creole seasoning, cover, and cook over medium-low heat for 30 minutes, or until the rice is tender. 5. Serve with a plate of greens of your choice.

Per Serving:

calorie: 274 | fat: 4g | protein: 16g | carbs: 43g | sugars: 2g | fiber: 3g | sodium: 79mg

Texas Caviar

Prep time: 10 minutes | Cook time: 0 minutes |
Serves 6

1 cup cooked black-eyed peas	½ red onion, chopped
1 cup cooked lima beans	3 tablespoons apple cider vinegar
1 ear fresh corn, kernels removed	2 tablespoons extra-virgin olive oil
2 celery stalks, chopped	1 teaspoon paprika
1 red bell pepper, chopped	

1. In a large bowl, combine the black-eyed peas, lima beans, corn, celery, bell pepper, and onion. 2. In a small bowl, to make the dressing, whisk the vinegar, oil, and paprika together. 3. Pour the dressing over the bean mixture, and gently mix. Set aside for 15 to 30 minutes, allowing the flavors to come together.

Per Serving:

calorie: 142 | fat: 5g | protein: 6g | carbs: 19g | sugars: 3g | fiber: 6g | sodium: 10mg

Sunshine Burgers

Prep time: 10 minutes | Cook time: 18 to 20 minutes | Makes 10 burgers

2 cups sliced raw carrots
1 large clove garlic, sliced or quartered
2 cans (15 ounces each) chickpeas, rinsed and drained
¼ cup sliced dry-packed sun-dried tomatoes
2 tablespoons tahini

1 teaspoon red wine vinegar or apple cider vinegar
1 teaspoon smoked paprika
½ teaspoon dried rosemary
½ teaspoon ground cumin
½ teaspoon sea salt
1 cup rolled oats

1. In a food processor, combine the carrots and garlic. Pulse several times to mince. Add the chickpeas, tomatoes, tahini, vinegar, paprika, rosemary, cumin, and salt. Puree until well combined, scraping down the sides of the bowl once or twice. Add the oats, and pulse briefly to combine. Refrigerate the mixture for 30 minutes, if possible. 2. Preheat the oven to 400°F. Line a baking sheet with parchment paper. 3. Use an ice cream scoop to scoop the mixture onto the prepared baking sheet, flattening to shape it into patties. Bake for 18 to 20 minutes, flipping the burgers halfway through. Alternatively, you can cook the burgers in a nonstick skillet over medium heat for 6 to 8 minutes Per side, or until golden brown. Serve.

Per Serving:
calorie: 137 | fat: 4 | protein: 6g | carbs: 21g | sugars: 4g | fiber: 6g | sodium: 278mg

Lentil Bolognese

Prep time: 10 minutes | Cook time: 30 minutes | Serves 4

⅓ cup red wine
1 cup diced onion
½ cup minced carrot
1 tablespoon dried oregano leaves
1 teaspoon vegan Worcestershire sauce
¾ teaspoon smoked paprika
½ teaspoon sea salt
¼ teaspoon ground nutmeg
1½ cups cooked brown or green

lentils
¼ cup chopped sun-dried tomatoes
1 can (28 ounces) diced tomatoes (use fire-roasted, if you'd like a spicy kick)
2 to 3 tablespoons minced dates
1 pound dry pasta
½ cup almond meal (toast until lightly golden if you want extra flavor)

1. In a large pot over high heat, combine the wine, onion, carrot, oregano, Worcestershire sauce, paprika, salt, and nutmeg. Cook for 5 minutes, stirring frequently. Add the lentils, sun-dried tomatoes, diced tomatoes, and dates, and bring to a boil. Reduce the heat to low, cover, and cook for 20 to 25 minutes. 2. While the sauce is simmering, prepare the pasta according to package directions. Once the pasta is almost cooked (still having some "bite," not mushy), drain and return it to the cooking pot. 3. Add the almond meal to the sauce, stir to incorporate, and cook for a couple of minutes.

Taste, season as desired, and toss with the pasta before serving.

Per Serving:
calorie: 754 | fat: 11g | protein: 31g | carbs: 132g | sugars: 14g | fiber: 17g | sodium: 622mg

Stewed Green Beans

Prep time: 5 minutes | Cook time: 10 minutes | Serves 4

1 pound green beans, trimmed
1 medium tomato, chopped
½ yellow onion, chopped
1 garlic clove, minced

1 teaspoon Creole seasoning
¼ cup store-bought low-sodium vegetable broth

1. In an electric pressure cooker, combine the green beans, tomato, onion, garlic, Creole seasoning, and broth. 2. Close and lock the lid, and set the pressure valve to sealing. 3. Select the Manual/Pressure Cook setting, and cook for 10 minutes. 4. Once cooking is complete, quick-release the pressure. Carefully remove the lid. 5. Transfer the beans to a serving dish. Serve warm.

Per Serving:
calorie: 58 | fat: 0g | protein: 3g | carbs: 13g | sugars: 7g | fiber: 4g | sodium: 98mg

Easy Lentil Burgers

Prep time: 10 minutes | Cook time: 20 minutes | Serves 5

1 medium-large clove garlic
2 tablespoons tamari
2 tablespoons tomato paste
1 tablespoon red wine vinegar
1½ tablespoons tahini
2 tablespoons fresh thyme or oregano

2 teaspoons onion powder
¼ teaspoon sea salt
Few pinches freshly ground black pepper
3 cups cooked brown lentils
1 cup toasted breadcrumbs
½ cup rolled oats

1. In a food processor, combine the garlic, tamari, tomato paste, vinegar, tahini, thyme or oregano, onion powder, salt, pepper, and 1½ cups of the lentils. Puree until fairly smooth. Add the breadcrumbs, rolled oats, and the remaining 1½ cups of lentils. Pulse a few times. At this stage you're looking for a sticky texture that will hold together when pressed. If the mixture is still a little crumbly, pulse a few more times. 2. Preheat the oven to 400°F. Line a baking sheet with parchment paper. 3. Use an ice cream scoop to scoop the mixture onto the prepared baking sheet, flattening to shape into patties. Bake for about 20 minutes, flipping the burgers halfway through. Alternatively, you can cook the burgers in a nonstick skillet over medium heat for 4 to 5 minutes Per side, or until golden brown.

Per Serving:
calorie: 148 | fat: 2g | protein: 8g | carbs: 24g | sugars: 1g | fiber: 5g | sodium: 369mg

Tex-Mex Rice 'N' Beans

Prep time: 10 minutes | Cook time: 25 minutes | Serves 4

1½ cups chopped bell pepper
1 to 1½ cups chopped onion
1 tablespoon dried oregano
2 teaspoons chili powder
½ tablespoon paprika
½ tablespoon ground cumin
1 teaspoon garlic powder
½ teaspoon cinnamon
Rounded ½ teaspoon sea salt

2 tablespoons water + 2½ cups water (boiled, if using an instant pot)
½ cup dried red lentils
1 cup uncooked brown rice (can substitute quinoa)
2 cans (15 ounces each) black beans, rinsed and drained
¼ cup tomato paste
1 bay leaf
2 tablespoons lime juice
Hot sauce to taste (optional)

1. In an instant pot, combine the bell pepper, onion, oregano, chili powder, paprika, cumin, garlic powder, cinnamon, salt, and 2 tablespoons of the water, and set to the sauté function. Cook for 3 to 4 minutes, stirring frequently. Turn off the sauté function and add the lentils, rice, beans, tomato paste, bay leaf, and the remaining 2½ cups water. Stir, cover the instant pot, and set to high pressure for 20 minutes. After 20 minutes, you can manually release the pressure or let it naturally release. Stir in the lime juice, taste, and season as desired. Add the hot sauce (if using), and serve.

Per Serving:

calorie: 525 | fat: 3g | protein: 24g | carbs: 103g | sugars: 7g | fiber: 25g | sodium: 898mg

Chapter 4 Beef, Pork, and Lamb

Goat Cheese-Stuffed Flank Steak

Prep time: 10 minutes | Cook time: 14 minutes | Serves 6

1 pound (454 g) flank steak	black pepper
1 tablespoon avocado oil	2 ounces (57 g) goat cheese,
½ teaspoon sea salt	crumbled
½ teaspoon garlic powder	1 cup baby spinach, chopped
¼ teaspoon freshly ground	

1. Place the steak in a large zip-top bag or between two pieces of plastic wrap. Using a meat mallet or heavy-bottomed skillet, pound the steak to an even ¼-inch thickness. 2. Brush both sides of the steak with the avocado oil. 3. Mix the salt, garlic powder, and pepper in a small dish. Sprinkle this mixture over both sides of the steak. 4. Sprinkle the goat cheese over top, and top that with the spinach. 5. Starting at one of the long sides, roll the steak up tightly. Tie the rolled steak with kitchen string at 3-inch intervals. 6. Set the air fryer to 400ºF (204ºC). Place the steak roll-up in the air fryer basket. Air fry for 7 minutes. Flip the steak and cook for an additional 7 minutes, until an instant-read thermometer reads 120ºF (49ºC) for medium-rare (adjust the cooking time for your desired doneness).

Per Serving:

calories: 151 | fat: 8g | protein: 18g | carbs: 0g | fiber: 0g | sodium: 281mg

Steaks with Walnut-Blue Cheese Butter

Prep time: 30 minutes | Cook time: 10 minutes | Serves 6

½ cup unsalted butter, at room temperature	1 teaspoon minced garlic
½ cup crumbled blue cheese	¼ teaspoon cayenne pepper
2 tablespoons finely chopped walnuts	Sea salt and freshly ground black pepper, to taste
1 tablespoon minced fresh rosemary	1½ pounds (680 g) New York strip steaks, at room temperature

1. In a medium bowl, combine the butter, blue cheese, walnuts, rosemary, garlic, and cayenne pepper and salt and black pepper to taste. Use clean hands to ensure that everything is well combined. Place the mixture on a sheet of parchment paper and form it into a log. Wrap it tightly in plastic wrap. Refrigerate for at least 2 hours or freeze for 30 minutes. 2. Season the steaks generously with salt and pepper. 3. Place the air fryer basket or grill pan in the air fryer.

Set the air fryer to 400ºF (204ºC) and let it preheat for 5 minutes. 4. Place the steaks in the basket in a single layer and air fry for 5 minutes. Flip the steaks, and cook for 5 minutes more, until an instant-read thermometer reads 120ºF (49ºC) for medium-rare (or as desired). 5. Transfer the steaks to a plate. Cut the butter into pieces and place the desired amount on top of the steaks. Tent a piece of aluminum foil over the steaks and allow to sit for 10 minutes before serving. 6. Store any remaining butter in a sealed container in the refrigerator for up to 2 weeks.

Per Serving:

calories: 283 | fat: 18g | protein: 30g | carbs: 1g | net carbs: 1g | fiber: 0g

Basic Nutritional Values

Prep time: 20 minutes | Cook time: 2 hours | Serves 4 to 6

2 pounds beef roast, boneless	2 cloves garlic, finely chopped,
¼ teaspoon salt	or 1 teaspoon garlic powder
¼ teaspoon pepper	1 teaspoon thyme
1 tablespoon olive oil	1 bay leaf
2 stalks celery, chopped	4 carrots, chopped
4 tablespoons margarine	1 medium onion, chopped
2 cups low-sodium tomato juice	4 medium potatoes, chopped

1. Pat beef dry with paper towels; season on all sides with salt and pepper. 2. Select Sauté function on the Instant Pot and adjust heat to more. Put the oil in the inner pot, then cook the beef in oil for 6 minutes, until browned, turning once. Set on plate. 3. Add celery and margarine to the inner pot; cook 2 minutes. Stir in tomato juice, garlic, thyme, and bay leaf. Hit Cancel to turn off Sauté function. 4. Place beef on top of the contents of the inner pot and press into sauce. Cover and lock lid and make sure vent is at sealing. Select Manual and cook at high pressure for 1 hour 15 minutes. 5. Once cooking is complete, release pressure by using natural release function. Transfer beef to cutting board. Discard bay leaf. 6. Skim off any excess fat from surface. Choose Sauté function and adjust heat to more. Cook 18 minutes, or until reduced by about half (2½ cups). Hit Cancel to turn off Sauté function. 7. Add carrots, onion, and potatoes. Cover and lock lid and make sure vent is at sealing. Select Manual and cook at high pressure for 10 minutes. 8. Once cooking is complete, release pressure by using a quick release. Using Sauté function, keep at a simmer. 9. Season with more salt and pepper to taste.

Per Serving:

calories: 391 | fat: 19 g | protein: 34g | carbs: 22g | sugars: 6g | fiber: 4g | sodium: 395mg

Sloppy Joes

Prep time: 10 minutes | Cook time: 15 minutes |
Serves 4

1 pound 93% lean ground beef
½ medium yellow onion, chopped
1 medium red bell pepper, chopped
1 (15 ounces) can no-salt-added tomato sauce

2 tablespoons no-salt-added, no-sugar-added ketchup
2 tablespoons low-sodium Worcestershire sauce
4 sandwich thins, 100% whole-wheat
1 cup shredded cabbage

1. Heat a large skillet over medium heat. When hot, cook the beef, onion, and bell pepper for 7 to 10 minutes, stirring and breaking apart as needed. 2. Stir in the tomato sauce, ketchup, and Worcestershire sauce. Increase the heat to medium-high and simmer for 5 minutes. 3. Cut the sandwich thins in half so there is a top and a bottom. For each serving, place one-quarter of the filling and cabbage on the bottom half, then cover with the top half.

Per Serving:

calorie: 309 | fat: 8g | protein: 30g | carbs: 33g | sugars: 11g | fiber: 6g | sodium: 368mg

Grilled Pork Loin Chops

Prep time: 15 minutes | Cook time: 30 minutes |
Serves 2

2 garlic cloves, minced
3 tablespoons Worcestershire sauce
2 tablespoons water
1 tablespoon low-sodium soy sauce
2 teaspoons tomato paste
1 teaspoon granulated stevia

½ teaspoon ground ginger
½ teaspoon onion powder
¼ teaspoon cinnamon
⅛ teaspoon cayenne pepper
2 (6 ounces) thick-cut boneless pork loin chops
Olive oil, for greasing the grill

1. In a small bowl, mix together the garlic, Worcestershire sauce, water, soy sauce, tomato paste, stevia, ginger, onion powder, cinnamon, and cayenne pepper. Pour half of the marinade into a large plastic sealable bag. Cover and refrigerate the remaining marinade. 2. Add the pork chops to the bag and seal. Refrigerate for 4 to 8 hours, turning occasionally. 3. Preheat the grill to medium. 4. With the olive oil, lightly oil the grill grate. 5. Remove the pork chops from the bag. Discard the marinade in the bag. 6. Place the chops on the preheated grill, basting with the remaining reserved half of the marinade. Grill for 8 to 12 minutes per side, or until the meat is browned, no longer pink inside, and an instant-read thermometer inserted into the thickest part of the chop reads at least 145°F. 7. In a saucepan set over medium heat, pour any remaining reserved marinade. Bring to a boil. Reduce the heat to low. Simmer for about 5 minutes, stirring constantly, until slightly thickened. 8. To serve, plate the chops and spoon the sauce over.

Per Serving:

calorie: 254 | fat: 6g | protein: 39g | carbs: 9g | sugars: 3g | fiber: 1g | sodium: 593mg

Easy Beef Curry

Prep time: 15 minutes | Cook time: 10 minutes |
Serves 6

1 tablespoon extra-virgin olive oil
1 small onion, thinly sliced
2 teaspoons minced fresh ginger
3 garlic cloves, minced
2 teaspoons ground coriander
1 teaspoon ground cumin
1 jalapeño or serrano pepper, slit lengthwise but not all the

way through
¼ teaspoon ground turmeric
¼ teaspoon salt
1 pound grass-fed sirloin tip steak, top round steak, or top sirloin steak, cut into bite-size pieces
2 tablespoons chopped fresh cilantro

1. In a large skillet, heat the oil over medium high. 2. Add the onion, and cook for 3 to 5 minutes until browned and softened. Add the ginger and garlic, stirring continuously until fragrant, about 30 seconds. 3. In a small bowl, mix the coriander, cumin, jalapeño, turmeric, and salt. Add the spice mixture to the skillet and stir continuously for 1 minute. Deglaze the skillet with about ¼ cup of water. 4. Add the beef and stir continuously for about 5 minutes until well-browned yet still medium rare. Remove the jalapeño. Serve topped with the cilantro.

Per Serving:

calories: 140 | fat: 7g | protein: 18g | carbs: 3g | sugars: 1g | fiber: 1g | sodium: 141mg

Rosemary Lamb Chops

Prep time: 25 minutes | Cook time: 2 minutes |
Serves 4

1½ pounds lamb chops (4 small chops)
1 teaspoon kosher salt
Leaves from 1 (6-inch) rosemary sprig

2 tablespoons avocado oil
1 shallot, peeled and cut in quarters
1 tablespoon tomato paste
1 cup beef broth

1. Place the lamb chops on a cutting board. Press the salt and rosemary leaves into both sides of the chops. Let rest at room temperature for 15 to 30 minutes. 2. Set the electric pressure cooker to Sauté/More setting. When hot, add the avocado oil. 3. Brown the lamb chops, about 2 minutes per side. (If they don't all fit in a single layer, brown them in batches.) 4. Transfer the chops to a plate. In the pot, combine the shallot, tomato paste, and broth. Cook for about a minute, scraping up the brown bits from the bottom. Hit Cancel. 5. Add the chops and any accumulated juices back to the pot. 6. Close and lock the lid of the pressure cooker. Set the valve to sealing. 7. Cook on high pressure for 2 minutes. 8. When the cooking is complete, hit Cancel and quick release the pressure. 9. Once the pin drops, unlock and remove the lid. 10. Place the lamb chops on plates and serve immediately.

Per Serving:

calorie: 352 | fat: 20g | protein: 37g | carbs: 7g | sugars: 1g | fiber: 0g | sodium: 440mg

Roasted Pork Loin

Prep time: 5 minutes | Cook time: 40 minutes |

Serves 4

1 pound pork loin
1 tablespoon extra-virgin olive oil, divided
2 teaspoons honey
¼ teaspoon freshly ground black pepper
½ teaspoon dried rosemary
2 small gold potatoes, chopped into 2-inch cubes
4 (6-inch) carrots, chopped into ½-inch rounds

1. Preheat the oven to 350°F. 2. Rub the pork loin with ½ tablespoon of oil and the honey. Season with the pepper and rosemary. 3. In a medium bowl, toss the potatoes and carrots in the remaining ½ tablespoon of oil. 4. Place the pork and the vegetables on a baking sheet in a single layer. Cook for 40 minutes. 5. Remove the baking sheet from the oven and let the pork rest for at least 10 minutes before slicing. Divide the pork and vegetables into four equal portions.

Per Serving:

calorie: 281 | fat: 8g | protein: 28g | carbs: 24g | sugars: 6g | fiber: 4g | sodium: 103mg

Sage-Parmesan Pork Chops

Prep time: 30 minutes | Cook time: 25 minutes |

Serves 2

Extra-virgin olive oil cooking spray
2 tablespoons coconut flour
¼ teaspoon salt
Pinch freshly ground black pepper
¼ cup almond meal
½ cup finely ground flaxseed meal
½ cup soy Parmesan cheese
1½ teaspoons rubbed sage
½ teaspoon grated lemon zest
2 (4 ounces) boneless pork chops
1 large egg, lightly beaten
1 tablespoon extra-virgin olive oil

1. Preheat the oven to 425°F. 2. Lightly coat a medium baking dish with cooking spray. 3. In a shallow dish, mix together the coconut flour, salt, and pepper. 4. In a second shallow dish, stir together the almond meal, flaxseed meal, soy Parmesan cheese, sage, and lemon zest. 5. Gently press one pork chop into the coconut flour mixture to coat. Shake off any excess. Dip into the beaten egg. Press into the almond meal mixture. Gently toss between your hands so any coating that hasn't stuck can fall away. Place the coated chop on a plate. Repeat the process with the remaining pork chop and coating ingredients. 6. In a large skillet set over medium heat, heat the olive oil. 7. Add the coated chops. Cook for about 4 minutes per side, or until browned. Transfer to the prepared baking dish. Place the dish in the preheated oven. Bake for 10 to 15 minutes, or until the juices run clear and an instant-read thermometer inserted into the middle of the pork reads 160°F.

Per Serving:

calorie: 520 | fat: 31g | protein: 45g | carbs: 14g | sugars: 1g | fiber: 6g | sodium: 403mg

Salisbury Steaks with Seared Cauliflower

Prep time: 5 minutes | Cook time: 30 minutes |

Serves 4

Salisbury Steaks
1 pound 95 percent lean ground beef
⅓ cup almond flour
1 large egg
½ teaspoon fine sea salt
¼ teaspoon freshly ground black pepper
2 tablespoons cold-pressed avocado oil
1 small yellow onion, sliced
1 garlic clove, chopped
8 ounces cremini or button mushrooms, sliced
½ teaspoon fine sea salt
2 tablespoons tomato paste
1½ teaspoons yellow mustard
1 cup low-sodium roasted beef bone broth
Seared Cauliflower
1 tablespoon olive oil
1 head cauliflower, cut into bite-size florets
2 tablespoons chopped fresh flat-leaf parsley
¼ teaspoon fine sea salt
2 teaspoons cornstarch
2 teaspoons water

1. To make the steaks: In a bowl, combine the beef, almond flour, egg, salt, and pepper and mix with your hands until all of the ingredients are evenly distributed. Divide the mixture into four equal portions, then shape each portion into an oval patty about ½ inch thick. 2. Select the Sauté setting on the Instant Pot and heat the oil for 2 minutes. Swirl the oil to coat the bottom of the pot, then add the patties and sear for 3 minutes, until browned on one side. Using a thin, flexible spatula, flip the patties and sear the second side for 2 to 3 minutes, until browned. Transfer the patties to a plate. 3. Add the onion, garlic, mushrooms, and salt to the pot and sauté for 4 minutes, until the onion is translucent and the mushrooms have begun to give up their liquid. Add the tomato paste, mustard, and broth and stir with a wooden spoon, using it to nudge any browned bits from the bottom of the pot. Return the patties to the pot in a single layer and spoon a bit of the sauce over each one. 4. Secure the lid and set the Pressure Release to Sealing. Press the Cancel button to reset the cooking program, then select the Pressure Cook or Manual setting and set the cooking time for 10 minutes at high pressure. (The pot will take about 5 minutes to come up to pressure before the cooking program begins.) 5. When the cooking program ends, let the pressure release naturally for at least 10 minutes, then move the Pressure Release to Venting to release any remaining steam. 6. To make the cauliflower: While the pressure is releasing, in a large skillet over medium heat, warm the oil. Add the cauliflower and stir or toss to coat with the oil, then cook, stirring every minute or two, until lightly browned, about 8 minutes. Turn off the heat, sprinkle in the parsley and salt, and stir to combine. Leave in the skillet, uncovered, to keep warm. 7. Open the pot and, using a slotted spatula, transfer the patties to a serving plate. In a small bowl, stir together the cornstarch and water. Press the Cancel button to reset the cooking program, then select the Sauté setting. When the sauce comes to a simmer, stir in the cornstarch mixture and let the sauce boil for about 1 minute, until thickened. Press the Cancel button to turn off the Instant Pot. 8. Spoon the sauce over the patties. Serve right away, with the cauliflower.

Per Serving:

calorie: 362 | fat: 21g | protein: 33g | carbs: 21g | sugars: 4g | fiber: 6g | sodium: 846mg

Beef Barley Soup

Prep time: 20 minutes | Cook time: 30 minutes |

Serves 4

2 teaspoons extra-virgin olive oil
1 sweet onion, chopped
1 tablespoon minced garlic
4 celery stalks, with greens, chopped
2 carrots, peeled, diced
1 sweet potato, peeled, diced
8 cups low-sodium beef broth

1 cup cooked pearl barley
2 cups diced cooked beef
2 bay leaves
2 teaspoons hot sauce
2 teaspoons chopped fresh thyme
1 cup shredded kale
Sea salt
Freshly ground black pepper

1. Place a large stockpot over medium-high heat and add the oil. 2. Sauté the onion and garlic until softened and translucent, about 3 minutes. 3. Stir in the celery, carrot, and sweet potato, and sauté for a further 5 minutes. 4. Stir in the beef broth, barley, beef, bay leaves, and hot sauce. 5. Bring the soup to a boil, then reduce the heat to low. 6. Simmer until the vegetables are tender, about 15 minutes. 7. Remove the bay leaves and stir in the thyme and kale. 8. Simmer for 5 minutes, and season with salt and pepper.

Per Serving:

calorie: 652 | fat: 22g | protein: 45g | carbs: 76g | sugars: 9g | fiber: 6g | sodium: 252mg

Fresh Pot Pork Butt

Prep time: 10 minutes | Cook time: 45 minutes |

Serves 8

2 tablespoons extra-virgin olive oil
¼ cup apple cider vinegar
1 tablespoon freshly ground black pepper
1 tablespoon dried oregano
1 small yellow onion, minced
2 scallions, white and green

parts, minced
1 celery stalk, minced
Juice of 1 lime
2 pounds boneless pork butt
4 garlic cloves, sliced
1 cup store-bought low-sodium chicken broth

1. In a medium bowl, combine the oil, vinegar, pepper, oregano, onion, scallions, celery, and lime juice. Mix well until a paste is formed. 2. Score the pork with 1-inch-deep cuts in a diamond pattern on both sides. Push the garlic into the slits. 3. Massage the paste all over meat. Cover and refrigerate overnight or for at least 4 hours. 4. Select the Sauté setting on an electric pressure cooker. Cook the meat for 2 minutes on each side. 5. Add the broth, close and lock the lid, and set the pressure valve to sealing. 6. Change to the Manual/Pressure Cook setting, and cook for 20 minutes. 7. Once cooking is complete, allow the pressure to release naturally. Carefully remove the lid. 8. Remove the pork from the pressure cooker, and serve.

Per Serving:

calorie: 197 | fat: 10g | protein: 22g | carbs: 3g | sugars: 1g | fiber: 1g | sodium: 86mg

Coffee-and-Herb-Marinated Steak

Prep time: 10 minutes | Cook time: 10 minutes |

Serves 4

¼ cup whole coffee beans
2 teaspoons minced garlic
2 teaspoons chopped fresh rosemary
2 teaspoons chopped fresh thyme
1 teaspoon freshly ground black

pepper
2 tablespoons apple cider vinegar
2 tablespoons extra-virgin olive oil
1 pound flank steak, trimmed of visible fat

1. Place the coffee beans, garlic, rosemary, thyme, and black pepper in a coffee grinder or food processor and pulse until coarsely ground. 2. Transfer the coffee mixture to a resealable plastic bag and add the vinegar and oil. Shake to combine. 3. Add the flank steak and squeeze the excess air out of the bag. Seal it. Marinate the steak in the refrigerator for at least 2 hours, occasionally turning the bag over. 4. Preheat the broiler. Line a baking sheet with aluminum foil. 5. Take the steak out of the bowl and discard the marinade. 6. Place the steak on the baking sheet and broil until it is done to your liking, about 5 minutes per side for medium. 7. Let the steak rest for 10 minutes before slicing it thinly on a bias. 8. Serve with a mixed green salad or your favorite side dish.

Per Serving:

calorie: 191 | fat: 9g | protein: 25g | carbs: 1g | sugars: 0g | fiber: 0g | sodium: 127mg

Quick Steak Tacos

Prep time: 5 minutes | Cook time: 10 minutes |

Serves 6

1 tablespoon olive oil
8 ounces sirloin steak
2 tablespoons steak seasoning
1 teaspoon Worcestershire sauce
½ red onion, halved and sliced
6 corn tortillas

¼ cup tomatoes
¾ cup reduced-fat Mexican cheese
2 tablespoons low-fat sour cream
6 tablespoons garden fresh salsa
¼ cup chopped fresh cilantro

1. Turn the Instant Pot on the Sauté function. When the pot displays "hot," add the olive oil to the pot. 2. Season the steak with the steak seasoning. 3. Add the steak to the pot along with the Worcestershire sauce. 4. Cook each side of the steak for 2–3 minutes until the steak turns brown. 5. Remove the steak from the pot and slice thinly. 6. Add the onion to the pot with the remaining olive oil and steak juices and cook them until translucent. 7. Remove the onion from the pot. 8. Warm your corn tortillas, then assemble your steak, onion, tomatoes, cheese, sour cream, salsa, and cilantro on top of each.

Per Serving:

calories: 187 | fat: 9g | protein: 14g | carbs: 14g | sugars: 2g | fiber: 2g | sodium: 254mg

Loaded Cottage Pie

Prep time: 15 minutes | Cook time: 1 hour | Serves 6 to 8

4 large russet potatoes, peeled and halved
3 tablespoons extra-virgin olive oil, divided
1 small onion, chopped
1 bunch collard greens, stemmed and thinly sliced
2 carrots, peeled and chopped
2 medium tomatoes, chopped
1 garlic clove, minced
1 pound 90 percent lean ground

beef
½ cup store-bought low-sodium chicken broth
1 teaspoon Worcestershire sauce
1 teaspoon celery seeds
1 teaspoon smoked paprika
½ teaspoon dried chives
½ teaspoon ground mustard
½ teaspoon cayenne pepper

1. Preheat the oven to 400°F. 2. Bring a large pot of water to a boil. 3. Add the potatoes, and boil for 15 to 20 minutes, or until fork-tender. 4. Transfer the potatoes to a large bowl and mash with 1 tablespoon of olive oil. 5. In a large cast iron skillet, heat the remaining 2 tablespoons of olive oil. 6. Add the onion, collard greens, carrots, tomatoes, and garlic and sauté, stirring often, for 7 to 10 minutes, or until the vegetables are softened. 7. Add the beef, broth, Worcestershire sauce, celery seeds, and smoked paprika. 8. Spread the meat and vegetable mixture evenly onto the bottom of a casserole dish. Sprinkle the chives, ground mustard, and cayenne on top of the mixture. Spread the mashed potatoes evenly over the top. 9. Transfer the casserole dish to the oven, and bake for 30 minutes, or until the top is light golden brown.

Per Serving:
calorie: 358 | fat: 10g | protein: 22g | carbs: 48g | sugars: 4g | fiber: 8g | sodium: 98mg

Lamb, Mushroom, and Goat Cheese Burgers

Prep time: 15 minutes | Cook time: 15 minutes | Serves 4

8 ounces grass-fed ground lamb
8 ounces brown mushrooms, finely chopped
¼ teaspoon salt

¼ teaspoon freshly ground black pepper
¼ cup crumbled goat cheese
1 tablespoon minced fresh basil

1. In a large mixing bowl, combine the lamb, mushrooms, salt, and pepper, and mix well. 2. In a small bowl, mix the goat cheese and basil. 3. Form the lamb mixture into 4 patties, reserving about ½ cup of the mixture in the bowl. In each patty, make an indentation in the center and fill with 1 tablespoon of the goat cheese mixture. Use the reserved meat mixture to close the burgers. Press the meat firmly to hold together. 4. Heat the barbecue or a large skillet over medium-high heat. Add the burgers and cook for 5 to 7 minutes on each side, until cooked through. Serve.

Per Serving:
calories: 173 | fat: 13g | protein: 11g | carbs: 3g | sugars: 1g | fiber: 0g | sodium: 154mg

Broiled Dijon Burgers

Prep time: 25 minutes | Cook time: 10 minutes | Makes 6 burgers

¼ cup fat-free egg product or 2 egg whites
2 tablespoons fat-free (skim) milk
2 teaspoons Dijon mustard or horseradish sauce
¼ teaspoon salt
⅛ teaspoon pepper

1 cup soft bread crumbs (about 2 slices bread)
1 small onion, finely chopped (⅓ cup)
1 pound extra-lean (at least 90%) ground beef
6 whole-grain burger buns, split, toasted

1 Set oven control to broil. Spray broiler pan rack with cooking spray. 2 In medium bowl, mix egg product, milk, mustard, salt and pepper. Stir in bread crumbs and onion. Stir in beef. Shape mixture into 6 patties, each about ½ inch thick. Place patties on rack in broiler pan. 3 Broil with tops of patties about 5 inches from heat 6 minutes. Turn; broil until meat thermometer inserted in center of patties reads 160°F, 4 to 6 minutes longer. Serve patties in buns.

Per Serving:
calories: 250 | fat: 8g | protein: 22g | carbs: 23g | sugars: 5g | fiber: 3g | sodium: 450mg

Chinese Spareribs

Prep time: 10 minutes | Cook time: 40 minutes | Serves 2

2 tablespoons hoisin sauce
2 tablespoons tomato paste
2 tablespoons water
1 tablespoon rice vinegar
2 teaspoons sesame oil
2 teaspoons low-sodium soy sauce
2 teaspoons Chinese five-spice

powder
2 garlic cloves, minced
1 teaspoon freshly squeezed lemon juice
1 teaspoon grated fresh ginger
½ teaspoon granulated stevia
1 pound pork spareribs

1. In a shallow glass dish, mix together the hoisin sauce, tomato paste, water, rice vinegar, sesame oil, soy sauce, Chinese five-spice powder, garlic, lemon juice, ginger, and stevia. 2. Add the ribs to the marinade. Turn to coat. Cover and refrigerate for 2 hours, or overnight. 3. Preheat the oven to 325°F. 4. Place a rack in the center of the oven. 5. Fill a broiler tray with enough water to cover the bottom. Place the grate over the tray. Arrange the ribs on the grate. Reserve the marinade. 6. Place the broiler pan in the preheated oven. Cook for 40 minutes, turning and brushing with the reserved marinade every 10 minutes. 7. Finish under the broiler for a crispier texture, if desired. Discard any remaining marinade. 8. Serve immediately with lots of napkins and enjoy!

Per Serving:
calorie: 594 | fat: 39g | protein: 45g | carbs: 13g | sugars: 8g | fiber: 1g | sodium: 557mg

Beef Burgundy

2 tablespoons olive oil
2 pounds stewing meat, cubed, trimmed of fat
2½ tablespoons flour
5 medium onions, thinly sliced
½ pound fresh mushrooms, sliced

1 teaspoon salt
¼ teaspoon dried marjoram
¼ teaspoon dried thyme
⅛ teaspoon pepper
¾ cup beef broth
1½ cups burgundy

1. Press Sauté on the Instant pot and add in the olive oil. 2. Dredge meat in flour, then brown in batches in the Instant Pot. Set aside the meat. Sauté the onions and mushrooms in the remaining oil and drippings for about 3–4 minutes, then add the meat back in. Press Cancel. 3. Add the salt, marjoram, thyme, pepper, broth, and wine to the Instant Pot. 4. Secure the lid and make sure the vent is set to sealing. Press the Manual button and set to 30 minutes. 5. When cook time is up, let the pressure release naturally for 15 minutes, then perform a quick release. 6. Serve over cooked noodles.

Per Serving:
calories: 358 | fat: 11g | protein: 37g | carbs: 15g | sugars: 5g | fiber: 2g | sodium: 472mg

Poblano Pepper Cheeseburgers

2 poblano chile peppers
1½ pounds (680 g) 85% lean ground beef
1 clove garlic, minced
1 teaspoon salt

½ teaspoon freshly ground black pepper
4 slices Cheddar cheese (about 3 ounces / 85 g)
4 large lettuce leaves

1. Preheat the air fryer to 400°F (204°C). 2. Arrange the poblano peppers in the basket of the air fryer. Pausing halfway through the cooking time to turn the peppers, air fry for 20 minutes, or until they are softened and beginning to char. Transfer the peppers to a large bowl and cover with a plate. When cool enough to handle, peel off the skin, remove the seeds and stems, and slice into strips. Set aside. 3. Meanwhile, in a large bowl, combine the ground beef with the garlic, salt, and pepper. Shape the beef into 4 patties. 4. Lower the heat on the air fryer to 360°F (182°C). Arrange the burgers in a single layer in the basket of the air fryer. Pausing halfway through the cooking time to turn the burgers, air fry for 10 minutes, or until a thermometer inserted into the thickest part registers 160°F (71°C). 5. Top the burgers with the cheese slices and continue baking for a minute or two, just until the cheese has melted. Serve the burgers on a lettuce leaf topped with the roasted poblano peppers.

Per Serving:
calories: 489 | fat: 35g | protein: 39g | carbs: 3g | fiber: 1g | sodium: 703mg

Pork Medallions with Cherry Sauce

1 pork tenderloin (1 to 1¼ pounds), cut into ½-inch slices
½ teaspoon garlic-pepper blend
2 teaspoons olive oil
¾ cup cherry preserves

2 tablespoons chopped shallots
1 tablespoon Dijon mustard
1 tablespoon balsamic vinegar
1 clove garlic, finely chopped

1. Sprinkle both sides of pork with garlic-pepper blend. 2. In 12-inch skillet, heat 1 teaspoon of the oil over medium-high heat. Add pork; cook 6 to 8 minutes, turning once, until pork is browned and meat thermometer inserted in center reads 145°F. Remove pork from skillet; keep warm. 3. In same skillet, mix remaining teaspoon oil, the preserves, shallots, mustard, vinegar and garlic, scraping any brown bits from bottom of skillet. Heat to boiling. Reduce heat; simmer uncovered 10 minutes or until reduced to about ½ cup. Serve sauce over pork slices.

Per Serving:
calorie: 330 | fat: 7g | protein: 23g | carbs: 44g | sugars: 30g | fiber: 1g | sodium: 170mg

Autumn Pork Chops with Red Cabbage and Apples

¼ cup apple cider vinegar
2 tablespoons granulated sweetener
4 (4 ounces) pork chops, about 1 inch thick
Sea salt
Freshly ground black pepper

1 tablespoon extra-virgin olive oil
½ red cabbage, finely shredded
1 sweet onion, thinly sliced
1 apple, peeled, cored, and sliced
1 teaspoon chopped fresh thyme

1. In a small bowl, whisk together the vinegar and sweetener. Set it aside. 2. Season the pork with salt and pepper. 3. Place a large skillet over medium-high heat and add the olive oil. 4. Cook the pork chops until no longer pink, turning once, about 8 minutes per side. 5. Transfer the chops to a plate and set aside. 6. Add the cabbage and onion to the skillet and sauté until the vegetables have softened, about 5 minutes. 7. Add the vinegar mixture and the apple slices to the skillet and bring the mixture to a boil. 8. Reduce the heat to low and simmer, covered, for 5 additional minutes. 9. Return the pork chops to the skillet, along with any accumulated juices and thyme, cover, and cook for 5 more minutes.

Per Serving:
calorie: 251 | fat: 8g | protein: 26g | carbs: 19g | sugars: 13g | fiber: 2g | sodium: 76mg

Easy Pot Roast and Vegetables

Prep time: 20 minutes | Cook time: 35 minutes | Serves 6

3 to 4 pounds chuck roast, trimmed of fat and cut into serving-sized chunks
4 medium potatoes, cubed, unpeeled

4 medium carrots, sliced, or 1 pound baby carrots
2 celery ribs, sliced thin
1 envelope dry onion soup mix
3 cups water

1. Place the pot roast chunks and vegetables into the Instant Pot along with the potatoes, carrots and celery. 2. Mix together the onion soup mix and water and pour over the contents of the Instant Pot. 3. Secure the lid and make sure the vent is set to sealing. Set the Instant Pot to Manual mode for 35 minutes. Let pressure release naturally when cook time is up.

Per Serving:

calorie: 325 | fat: 8g | protein: 35g | carbs: 26g | sugars: 6g | fiber: 4g | sodium: 560mg

Carnitas Burrito Bowls

Prep time: 10 minutes | Cook time: 1 hour | Serves 6

Carnitas
1 tablespoon chili powder
½ teaspoon garlic powder
1 teaspoon ground coriander
1 teaspoon fine sea salt
½ cup water
¼ cup fresh lime juice
One 2 pounds boneless pork shoulder butt roast, cut into 2-inch cubes
Rice and Beans
1 cup Minute brand brown rice (see Note)
1½ cups drained cooked black beans, or one 15 ounces can black beans, rinsed and drained
Pico de Gallo
8 ounces tomatoes (see Note),

diced
½ small yellow onion, diced
1 jalapeño chile, seeded and finely diced
1 tablespoon chopped fresh cilantro
1 teaspoon fresh lime juice
Pinch of fine sea salt
¼ cup sliced green onions, white and green parts
2 tablespoons chopped fresh cilantro
3 hearts romaine lettuce, cut into ¼-inch-wide ribbons
2 large avocados, pitted, peeled, and sliced
Hot sauce (such as Cholula or Tapatío) for serving

1. To make the carnitas: In a small bowl, combine the chili powder, garlic powder, coriander, and salt and mix well. 2. Pour the water and lime juice into the Instant Pot. Add the pork, arranging the pieces in a single layer. Sprinkle the chili powder mixture evenly over the pork. 3. Secure the lid and set the Pressure Release to Sealing. Select the Meat/Stew setting and set the cooking time for 30 minutes at high pressure. (The pot will take about 10 minutes to come up to pressure before the cooking program begins.) 4. When the cooking program ends, let the pressure release naturally for at least 15 minutes, then move the Pressure Release to Venting to release any remaining steam. Open the pot and, using tongs, transfer the pork to a plate or cutting board. 5. While the pressure is releasing, preheat the oven to 400°F. 6. Wearing heat-resistant

mitts, lift out the inner pot and pour the cooking liquid into a fat separator. Pour the defatted cooking liquid into a liquid measuring cup and discard the fat. (Alternatively, use a ladle or large spoon to skim the fat off the surface of the liquid.) Add water as needed to the cooking liquid to total 1 cup (you may have enough without adding water). 7. To make the rice and beans: Pour the 1 cup cooking liquid into the Instant Pot and add the rice, making sure it is in an even layer. Place a tall steam rack into the pot. Add the black beans to a 1½-quart stainless-steel bowl and place the bowl on top of the rack. (The bowl should not touch the lid once the pot is closed.) 8. Secure the lid and set the Pressure Release to Sealing. Press the Cancel button to reset the cooking program, then select the Pressure Cook or Manual setting and set the cooking time for 15 minutes at high pressure. (The pot will take about 5 minutes to come to pressure before the cooking program begins.) 9. While the rice and beans are cooking, using two forks, shred the meat into bite-size pieces. Transfer the pork to a sheet pan, spreading it out in an even layer. Place in the oven for 20 minutes, until crispy and browned. 10. To make the pico de gallo: While the carnitas, rice, and beans are cooking, in a medium bowl, combine the tomatoes, onion, jalapeño, cilantro, lime juice, and salt and mix well. Set aside. 11. When the cooking program ends, let the pressure release naturally for 5 minutes, then move the Pressure Release to Venting to release any remaining steam. Open the pot and, wearing heat-resistant mitts, remove the bowl of beans and then the steam rack from the pot. Then remove the inner pot. Add the green onions and cilantro to the rice and, using a fork, fluff the rice and mix in the green onions and cilantro. 12. Divide the rice, beans, carnitas, pico de gallo, lettuce, and avocados evenly among six bowls. Serve warm, with the hot sauce on the side.

Per Serving:

calories: 447 | fat: 20g | protein: 31g | carbs: 35g | sugars: 4g | fiber: 9g | sodium: 653mg

Marjoram-Pepper Steaks

Prep time: 5 minutes | Cook time: 8 minutes | Serves 2

1 tablespoon freshly ground black pepper
¼ teaspoon dried marjoram
2 (6 ounces, 1-inch-thick) beef tenderloins

1 tablespoon extra-virgin olive oil
¼ cup low-sodium beef broth
Fresh marjoram sprigs, for garnish

1. In a large bowl, mix together the pepper and marjoram. 2. Add the steaks. Coat both sides with the spice mixture. 3. In a skillet set over medium-high heat, heat the olive oil. 4. Add the steaks. Cook for 5 to 7 minutes, or until an instant-read thermometer inserted in the center registers 160°F (for medium). Remove from the skillet. Cover to keep warm. 5. Add the broth to the skillet. Increase the heat to high. Bring to a boil, scraping any browned bits from the bottom. Boil for about 1 minute, or until the liquid is reduced by half. 6. Spoon the broth sauce over the steaks. Garnish with marjoram sprigs and serve immediately.

Per Serving:

calorie: 339 | fat: 19g | protein: 38g | carbs: 2g | sugars: 0g | fiber: 1g | sodium: 209mg

Roasted Beef with Peppercorn Sauce

Prep time: 10 minutes | Cook time:1hour | Serves 4

1½ pounds top rump beef roast
Sea salt
Freshly ground black pepper
3 teaspoons extra-virgin olive oil, divided
3 shallots, minced

2 teaspoons minced garlic
1 tablespoon green peppercorns
2 tablespoons dry sherry
2 tablespoons all-purpose flour
1 cup sodium-free beef broth

1. Heat the oven to 300°F. 2. Season the roast with salt and pepper. 3. Place a large skillet over medium-high heat and add 2 teaspoons of olive oil. 4. Brown the beef on all sides, about 10 minutes in total, and transfer the roast to a baking dish. 5. Roast until desired doneness, about 1½ hours for medium. When the roast has been in the oven for 1 hour, start the sauce. 6. In a medium saucepan over medium-high heat, sauté the shallots in the remaining 1 teaspoon of olive oil until translucent, about 4 minutes. 7. Stir in the garlic and peppercorns, and cook for another minute. Whisk in the sherry to deglaze the pan. 8. Whisk in the flour to form a thick paste, cooking for 1 minute and stirring constantly. 9. Pour in the beef broth and whisk until the sauce is thick and glossy, about 4 minutes. Season the sauce with salt and pepper. 10. Serve the beef with a generous spoonful of sauce.

Per Serving:

calorie: 272 | fat: 10g | protein: 40g | carbs: g | sugars: 0g | fiber: 0g | sodium: 331mg

Pork Mole Quesadillas

Prep time: 35 minutes | Cook time: 15 minutes |

Makes 4 quesadillas

2 teaspoons canola oil
½ lb boneless pork loin chops, trimmed of fat, cut into thin strips
1 medium green bell pepper, thinly sliced
1 medium red bell pepper, thinly sliced
1 medium onion, thinly sliced
3 cloves garlic, finely chopped
1 tablespoon chili powder
1 teaspoon all-purpose flour
1 teaspoon ground cumin
¼ teaspoon salt

¼ teaspoon ground cinnamon
¼ cup reduced-sodium chicken broth
2 tablespoons semisweet chocolate chips
4 fat-free flour tortillas (10 inch)
Cooking spray
½ cup chopped tomato
4 teaspoons chopped fresh cilantro
½ cup shredded reduced-fat Monterey Jack cheese (2 ounces)

1 In 12-inch nonstick skillet, heat 1 teaspoon of the oil over medium-high heat. Add pork to oil. Cook 4 to 5 minutes, stirring frequently, until pork is no longer pink; remove from skillet. 2 In same skillet, heat remaining 1 teaspoon oil over medium heat. Add bell peppers, onion and garlic to oil. Cook 3 to 5 minutes, stirring occasionally, until bell peppers are crisp-tender. Stir in chili powder, flour, cumin, salt and cinnamon; cook 30 seconds. Stir in chicken broth; heat to boiling. Cook about 30 seconds, stirring constantly, until thickened and bubbly. Remove from heat; stir in chocolate chips until melted. Stir in pork. 3 Spray 1 side of each tortilla with cooking spray. On work surface, place tortillas, sprayed side down. Arrange pork mixture, tomato, cilantro and cheese evenly over half of each tortilla. Fold tortilla over filling, pressing gently. 4 Heat 12-inch skillet over medium heat until hot. Cook 2 quesadillas 3 to 4 minutes, turning once, until tortillas begin to brown; remove quesadillas from pan. Keep warm. Repeat with remaining 2 quesadillas. 5 To serve, cut into wedges, beginning from center of folded side.

Per Serving:

1 Quesadilla: calories: 450 | fat: 17g | protein: 23g | carbs: 50g | sugars: 8g | fiber: 4g | sodium: 810mg

Spiced Lamb Stew

Prep time: 20 minutes | Cook time: 2 hours | Serves 4

2 tablespoons extra-virgin olive oil
1½ pounds lamb shoulder, cut into 1-inch chunks
½ sweet onion, chopped
1 tablespoon grated fresh ginger
2 teaspoons minced garlic
1 teaspoon ground cinnamon

1 teaspoon ground cumin
¼ teaspoon ground cloves
2 sweet potatoes, peeled, diced
2 cups low-sodium beef broth
Sea salt
Freshly ground back pepper
2 teaspoons chopped fresh parsley, for garnish

1. Preheat the oven to 300°F. 2. Place a large ovenproof skillet over medium-high heat and add the olive oil. 3. Brown the lamb, stirring occasionally, for about 6 minutes. 4. Add the onion, ginger, garlic, cinnamon, cumin, and cloves, and sauté for 5 minutes. 5. Add the sweet potatoes and beef broth and bring the stew to a boil. 6. Cover the skillet and transfer the lamb to the oven. Braise, stirring occasionally, until the lamb is very tender, about 2 hours. 7. Remove the stew from the oven and season with salt and pepper. 8. Serve garnished with the parsley.

Per Serving:

calorie: 406 | fat: 21g | protein: 37g | carbs: 18g | sugars: 5g | fiber: 3g | sodium: 511mg

Mustard-Glazed Pork Chops

Prep time: 5 minutes | Cook time: 25 minutes |

Serves 4

¼ cup Dijon mustard
1 tablespoon pure maple syrup

2 tablespoons rice vinegar
4 bone-in, thin-cut pork chops

1. Preheat the oven to 400°F. 2. In a small saucepan, combine the mustard, maple syrup, and rice vinegar. Stir to mix and bring to a simmer over medium heat. Cook for about 2 minutes until just slightly thickened. 3. In a baking dish, place the pork chops and spoon the sauce over them, flipping to coat. 4. Bake, uncovered, for 18 to 22 minutes until the juices run clear.

Per Serving:

calories: 257 | fat: 7g | protein: 39g | carbs: 7g | sugars: 4g | fiber: 0g | sodium: 466mg

Traditional Beef Stroganoff

Prep time: 10 minutes | Cook time: 30 minutes | Serves 4

1 teaspoon extra-virgin olive oil	½ cup low-sodium beef broth
1 pound top sirloin, cut into thin strips	¼ cup dry sherry
1 cup sliced button mushrooms	½ cup fat-free sour cream
½ sweet onion, finely chopped	1 tablespoon chopped fresh parsley
1 teaspoon minced garlic	Sea salt
1 tablespoon whole-wheat flour	Freshly ground black pepper

1. Place a large skillet over medium-high heat and add the oil. 2. Sauté the beef until browned, about 10 minutes, then remove the beef with a slotted spoon to a plate and set it aside. 3. Add the mushrooms, onion, and garlic to the skillet and sauté until lightly browned, about 5 minutes. 4. Whisk in the flour and then whisk in the beef broth and sherry. 5. Return the sirloin to the skillet and bring the mixture to a boil. 6. Reduce the heat to low and simmer until the beef is tender, about 10 minutes. 7. Stir in the sour cream and parsley. Season with salt and pepper.

Per Serving:

calorie: 320 | fat: 18g | protein: 26g | carbs: 13g | sugars: 3g | fiber: 1g | sodium: 111mg

Pork Tacos

Prep time: 30 minutes | Cook time: 10 minutes | Serves 2

8 ounces boneless skinless pork tenderloin, thinly sliced, ¼-inch thick, across the grain	juice
	2 (6-inch) soft low-carb corn tortillas, such as La Tortilla
Pinch salt	4 tablespoons diced tomatoes, divided
⅓ cup ancho chile sauce	
2 tablespoons chipotle purée (see Recipe Tip)	1 cup shredded lettuce, divided
¼ cup freshly squeezed lime	½ avocado, sliced
	4 tablespoons salsa, divided

1. Sprinkle the pork slices with salt. Set aside. 2. In a small bowl, stir together the ancho chile sauce, chipotle purée, and lime juice. Reserve 3 tablespoons of the marinade. Set aside. 3. In a large sealable plastic bag, add the pork. Pour the remaining marinade over it. Seal the bag, removing as much air as possible. Marinate the meat for 20 minutes to 1 hour at room temperature, or refrigerate for several hours. Turn the meat twice while it marinates. 4. Place a small nonstick skillet over medium heat. Have a large piece of aluminum foil nearby. 5. Working with one tortilla at a time, heat both sides in the skillet until they puff slightly. As they are done, stack the tortillas on the foil. When they are all heated, wrap the tortillas in the foil. 6. Preheat the broiler. 7. Adjust the rack so it is 4 inches from the heating element. 8. Remove the pork slices from the marinade. Discard the marinade. Place the pork on a rack set over a sheet pan. 9. Place the pan in the oven. Broil for 3 to 4 minutes, or until the edges of the pork begin to brown. Remove from the oven. Turn and brush the pork with the reserved marinade. Broil the second side for 3 minutes, or until the pork is just barely pink inside. 10. Place the foil packet with the tortillas in the oven to warm while the pork finishes cooking. 11. To serve, pile each tortilla with a few slices of pork. Top each with about 2 tablespoons of diced tomato, ½ cup of shredded lettuce, half of the avocado slices, and about 2 tablespoons of salsa.

Per Serving:

calorie: 328 | fat: 13g | protein: 30g | carbs: 25g | sugars: 5g | fiber: 7g | sodium: 563mg

Spice-Rubbed Pork Loin

Prep time: 5 minutes | Cook time: 20 minutes | Serves 6

1 teaspoon paprika	1 (1½-pound / 680-g) boneless pork loin
½ teaspoon ground cumin	
½ teaspoon chili powder	½ teaspoon salt
½ teaspoon garlic powder	¼ teaspoon ground black pepper
2 tablespoons coconut oil	

1. In a small bowl, mix paprika, cumin, chili powder, and garlic powder. 2. Drizzle coconut oil over pork. Sprinkle pork loin with salt and pepper, then rub spice mixture evenly on all sides. 3. Place pork loin into ungreased air fryer basket. Adjust the temperature to 400ºF (204ºC) and air fry for 20 minutes, turning pork halfway through cooking. Pork loin will be browned and have an internal temperature of at least 145ºF (63ºC) when done. Serve warm.

Per Serving:

calories: 192 | fat: 9g | protein: 26g | carbs: 1g | fiber: 0g | sodium: 257mg

Pot Roast with Gravy and Vegetables

Prep time: 30 minutes | Cook time: 1 hour 15 minutes | Serves 6

1 tablespoon olive oil	or gravy browning seasoning sauce
3 to 4 pounds bottom round, rump, or arm roast, trimmed of fat	1 garlic clove, minced
	2 medium onions, cut in wedges
¼ teaspoon salt	4 medium potatoes, cubed, unpeeled
2 to 3 teaspoons pepper	
2 tablespoons flour	2 carrots, quartered
1 cup cold water	1 green bell pepper, sliced
1 teaspoon Kitchen Bouquet,	

1. Press the Sauté button on the Instant Pot and pour the oil inside, letting it heat up. Sprinkle each side of the roast with salt and pepper, then brown it for 5 minutes on each side inside the pot. 2. Mix together the flour, water and Kitchen Bouquet and spread over roast. 3. Add garlic, onions, potatoes, carrots, and green pepper. 4. Secure the lid and make sure the vent is set to sealing. Press Manual and set the Instant Pot for 1 hour and 15 minutes. 5. When cook time is up, let the pressure release naturally.

Per Serving:

calories: 551 | fat: 30g | protein: 49g | carbs: 19g | sugars: 2g | fiber: 3g | sodium: 256mg

Slow Cooker Ropa Vieja

Prep time: 5 minutes | Cook time: 20 minutes | Serves 4

½ small yellow onion
1 red bell pepper
1 (14 ounces) can no-salt-added diced tomatoes
1 teaspoon dried oregano
½ teaspoon salt

½ teaspoon smoked paprika
½ teaspoon garlic powder
1 pound chuck beef roast, trimmed of visible fat
1 head cauliflower

1. Cut the onion and bell pepper into ½-inch-thick slices. 2. Place the onion, bell pepper, diced tomatoes with their juices, oregano, salt, paprika, and garlic powder in a slow cooker, then add the beef. 3. Place the head of cauliflower on top of the beef, and cook on low for 8 hours. 4. When fully cooked, the cauliflower will fall apart when scooped.

Per Serving:

calorie: 228 | fat: 7g | protein: 27g | carbs: 14g | sugars: 7g | fiber: 6g | sodium: 445mg

Italian Beef Kebabs

Prep time: 25 minutes | Cook time: 10 minutes | Serves 2

2 garlic cloves, finely chopped
¼ cup balsamic vinegar
¼ cup water
2 tablespoons extra-virgin olive oil
1 tablespoon chopped fresh oregano leaves, or 1 teaspoon dried
1½ teaspoons chopped fresh marjoram leaves, or ½ teaspoon dried
1 teaspoon granulated stevia

1 (¾-pound, 1-inch-thick) beef bone-in sirloin, or round steak, fat removed, cut into 1-inch pieces
1 medium yellow squash, sliced
1 medium green bell pepper, cut into 1-inch squares
6 whole fresh button mushrooms
1 small red onion, cut into 1-inch squares

1. In a medium glass bowl, mix together the garlic, balsamic vinegar, water, olive oil, oregano, marjoram, and stevia. 2. Add the beef. Stir until coated. Cover and refrigerate, stirring occasionally, for at least 1 hour but no longer than 12 hours. 3. Preheat the oven to broil. 4. Remove the beef from the marinade, reserving the marinade. 5. Using 10-inch metal skewers, thread on 1 piece of beef, 1 piece of yellow squash, 1 piece of bell pepper, 1 mushroom, and 1 piece of onion, leaving ½ inch of space between each piece. Repeat with the remaining ingredients until all are used. Brush the kebabs with the reserved marinade. 6. Place the kebabs on a rack in the broiler pan. Place the pan under the preheated broiler about 3 inches from the heat. Broil for 6 to 8 minutes for medium-rare to medium doneness, turning and brushing with the marinade after 3 minutes. Discard any remaining marinade. 7. Enjoy this delightful meal on a stick!

Per Serving:

calorie: 494 | fat: 28g | protein: 42g | carbs: 19g | sugars: 11g | fiber: 4g | sodium: 114mg

Zoodles Carbonara

Prep time: 10 minutes | Cook time: 25 minutes | Serves 4

6 slices bacon, cut into pieces
1 red onion, finely chopped
3 zucchini, cut into noodles
1 cup peas
½ teaspoon sea salt
3 garlic cloves, minced

3 large eggs, beaten
1 tablespoon heavy cream
Pinch red pepper flakes
½ cup grated Parmesan cheese (optional, for garnish)

1. In a large skillet over medium-high heat, cook the bacon until browned, about 5 minutes. With a slotted spoon, transfer the bacon to a plate. 2. Add the onion to the bacon fat in the pan and cook, stirring, until soft, 3 to 5 minutes. Add the zucchini, peas, and salt. Cook, stirring, until the zucchini softens, about 3 minutes. Add the garlic and cook, stirring constantly, for 5 minutes. 3. In a small bowl, whisk together the eggs, cream, and red pepper flakes. Add to the vegetables. 4. Remove the pan from the stove top and stir for 3 minutes, allowing the heat of the pan to cook the eggs without setting them. 5. Return the bacon to the pan and stir to mix. 6. Serve topped with Parmesan cheese, if desired.

Per Serving:

calorie: 294 | fat: 21g | protein: 14g | carbs: 14g | sugars: 7g | fiber: 4g | sodium: 544mg

Mango-Glazed Pork Tenderloin Roast

Prep time: 10 minutes | Cook time: 20 minutes | Serves 4

1 pound boneless pork tenderloin, trimmed of fat
1 teaspoon chopped fresh rosemary
1 teaspoon chopped fresh thyme
¼ teaspoon salt, divided
¼ teaspoon freshly ground black pepper, divided

1 teaspoon extra-virgin olive oil
1 tablespoon honey
2 tablespoons white wine vinegar
2 tablespoons dry cooking wine
1 tablespoon minced fresh ginger
1 cup diced mango

1. Preheat the oven to 400°F. 2. Season the tenderloin with the rosemary, thyme, ⅛ teaspoon of salt, and ⅛ teaspoon of pepper. 3. Heat the olive oil in an oven-safe skillet over medium-high heat, and sear the tenderloin until browned on all sides, about 5 minutes total. 4. Transfer the skillet to the oven and roast for 12 to 15 minutes until the pork is cooked through, the juices run clear, and the internal temperature reaches 145°F. Transfer to a cutting board to rest for 5 minutes. 5. In a small bowl, combine the honey, vinegar, cooking wine, and ginger. In to the same skillet, pour the honey mixture and simmer for 1 minute. Add the mango and toss to coat. Transfer to a blender and purée until smooth. Season with the remaining ⅛ teaspoon of salt and ⅛ teaspoon of pepper. 6. Slice the pork into rounds and serve with the mango sauce.

Per Serving:

calories: 182 | fat: 4g | protein: 24 | carbs: 12g | sugars: 10g | fiber: 1g | sodium: 240mg

Herb-Marinated Tenderloins

Prep time: 30 minutes | Cook time: 20 minutes |
Serves 2

1 (8 ounces) beef tenderloin filet	pepper
6 fresh sage leaves	1 medium sweet potato
1 garlic clove, sliced into 6 pieces	12 cherry tomatoes, chopped
4 fresh rosemary sprigs	1 tablespoon finely chopped fresh chives
Dash salt	2 teaspoons extra-virgin olive oil
Dash freshly ground black	4 cups baby spinach, divided

1. Cut 3 (2-inch-deep) slits in each side of the filet. Stuff 1 sage leave and 1 garlic slice into each slit. Wrap the rosemary sprigs around the filet. Season with salt and pepper. Refrigerate for 12 hours, or overnight, to allow the meat to absorb the seasoning flavors. 2. The next day, preheat the broiler to high. 3. Drain the steak. Place on an unheated rack in the broiler pan. Place the pan in the preheated oven. Broil the steak for 13 to 17 minutes for medium (160°F), 3 inches from the heat, turning once halfway through. Remove from the oven. Let the filet rest for 2 to 3 minutes before cutting in half. Tent with aluminum foil to keep warm. 4. While the filet cooks, poke the sweet potato all over with a fork. Microwave on high for about 6 minutes, or until soft. Thinly slice the cooked potato into rounds. Keep warm. 5. In a small bowl, mix together the tomatoes, chives, and olive oil. 6. Place 2 cups of spinach on each serving plate. Arrange half of the sweet potato slices in a half-moon shape on each plate. Spoon half of the tomatoes over the sweet potatoes. Place 1 filet half in the center of each plate. 7. Enjoy!

Per Serving:
calorie: 318 | fat: 13g | protein: 29g | carbs: 21g | sugars: 6g | fiber: 6g | sodium: 231mg

Herb-Crusted Lamb Chops

Prep time: 10 minutes | Cook time: 5 minutes |
Serves 2

1 large egg	leaves
2 cloves garlic, minced	½ teaspoon ground black pepper
¼ cup pork dust	4 (1-inch-thick) lamb chops
¼ cup powdered Parmesan cheese	For Garnish/Serving (Optional):
1 tablespoon chopped fresh oregano leaves	Sprigs of fresh oregano
	Sprigs of fresh rosemary
1 tablespoon chopped fresh rosemary leaves	Sprigs of fresh thyme
	Lavender flowers
1 teaspoon chopped fresh thyme	Lemon slices

1. Spray the air fryer basket with avocado oil. Preheat the air fryer to 400°F (204°C). 2. Beat the egg in a shallow bowl, add the garlic, and stir well to combine. In another shallow bowl, mix together the pork dust, Parmesan, herbs, and pepper. 3. One at a time, dip the lamb chops into the egg mixture, shake off the excess egg, and then dredge them in the Parmesan mixture. Use your hands to coat the chops well in the Parmesan mixture and form a nice crust on all sides; if necessary, dip the chops again in both the egg and the Parmesan mixture. 4. Place the lamb chops in the air fryer basket, leaving space between them, and air fry for 5 minutes, or until the internal temperature reaches 145°F (63°C) for medium doneness. Allow to rest for 10 minutes before serving. 5. Garnish with sprigs of oregano, rosemary, and thyme, and lavender flowers, if desired. Serve with lemon slices, if desired. 6. Best served fresh. Store leftovers in an airtight container in the fridge for up to 4 days. Serve chilled over a salad, or reheat in a 350°F (177°C) air fryer for 3 minutes, or until heated through.

Per Serving:
calories: 510 | fat: 42g | protein: 30g | carbs: 3g | fiber: 1g | sodium: 380mg

Pork Carnitas

Prep time: 10 minutes | Cook time: 20 minutes |
Serves 8

1 teaspoon kosher salt	Juice and zest of 1 large orange
2 teaspoons chili powder	Juice and zest of 1 medium lime
2 teaspoons dried oregano	
½ teaspoon freshly ground black pepper	6-inch gluten-free corn tortillas, warmed, for serving (optional)
1 (2½ pounds) pork sirloin roast or boneless pork butt, cut into 1½-inch cubes	Chopped avocado, for serving (optional)
2 tablespoons avocado oil, divided	Roasted Tomatillo Salsa or salsa verde, for serving (optional)
3 garlic cloves, minced	Shredded cheddar cheese, for serving (optional)

1. In a large bowl or gallon-size zip-top bag, combine the salt, chili powder, oregano, and pepper. Add the pork cubes and toss to coat. 2. Set the electric pressure cooker to the Sauté/More setting. When the pot is hot, pour in 1 tablespoon of avocado oil. 3. Add half of the pork to the pot and sear until the pork is browned on all sides, about 5 minutes. Transfer the pork to a plate, add the remaining 1 tablespoon of avocado oil to the pot, and sear the remaining pork. Hit Cancel. 4. Return all of the pork to the pot and add the garlic, orange zest and juice, and lime zest and juice to the pot. 5. Close and lock the lid of the pressure cooker. Set the valve to sealing. 6. Cook on high pressure for 20 minutes. 7. When the cooking is complete, hit Cancel. Allow the pressure to release naturally for 15 minutes then quick release any remaining pressure. 8. Once the pin drops, unlock and remove the lid. 9. Using two forks, shred the meat right in the pot. 10. (Optional) For more authentic carnitas, spread the shredded meat on a broiler-safe sheet pan. Preheat the broiler with the rack 6 inches from the heating element. Broil the pork for about 5 minutes or until it begins to crisp. (Watch carefully so you don't let the pork burn.) 11. Place the pork in a serving bowl. Top with some of the juices from the pot. Serve with tortillas, avocado, salsa, and Cheddar cheese (if using).

Per Serving:
calorie: 218 | fat: 7g | protein: 33g | carbs: 4g | sugars: 2g | fiber: 1g | sodium: 400mg

Chapter 5 Poultry

Chicken Reuben Bake

Prep time: 10 minutes | Cook time: 6 to 8 hours |

Serves 6

4 boneless, skinless chicken-breast halves	Swiss cheese
¼ cup water	¾ cup fat-free Thousand Island salad dressing
1 pound bag sauerkraut, drained and rinsed	2 tablespoons chopped fresh parsley
4 to 5 (1 ounce each) slices	

1. Place chicken and water in inner pot of the Instant Pot along with ¼ cup water. Layer sauerkraut over chicken. Add cheese. Top with salad dressing. Sprinkle with parsley. 2. Secure the lid and cook on the Slow Cook setting on low 6–8 hours.

Per Serving:

calories: 217 | fat: 5g | protein: 28g | carbs: 13g | sugars: 6g | fiber: 2g | sodium: 693mg

Chicken with Creamy Thyme Sauce

Prep time: 15 minutes | Cook time: 30 minutes |

Serves 4

4 (4 ounces) boneless, skinless chicken breasts	broth
Sea salt	2 teaspoons chopped fresh thyme
Freshly ground black pepper	¼ cup heavy (whipping) cream
1 tablespoon extra-virgin olive oil	1 tablespoon butter
½ sweet onion, chopped	1 scallion, white and green parts, chopped
1 cup low-sodium chicken	

1. Preheat the oven to 375°F. 2. Season the chicken breasts lightly with salt and pepper. 3. Place a large ovenproof skillet over medium-high heat and add the olive oil. 4. Brown the chicken, turning once, about 10 minutes in total. Transfer the chicken to a plate. 5. In the same skillet, sauté the onion until softened and translucent, about 3 minutes. 6. Add the chicken broth and thyme, and simmer until the liquid has reduced by half, about 6 minutes. 7. Stir in the cream and butter, and return the chicken and any accumulated juices from the plate to the skillet. 8. Transfer the skillet to the oven. Bake until cooked through, about 10 minutes. 9. Serve topped with the chopped scallion.

Per Serving:

calorie: 240 | fat: 12g | protein: 27g | carbs: 4g | sugars: 2g | fiber: 0g | sodium: 231mg

Grilled Lemon Mustard Chicken

Prep time: 5 minutes | Cook time: 15 minutes |

Serves 6

Juice of 6 medium lemons	4 garlic cloves, minced
½ cup mustard seeds	2 tablespoons extra-virgin olive oil
1 tablespoon minced fresh tarragon	Three 8 ounces boneless, skinless chicken breasts, halved
2 tablespoons freshly ground black pepper	

1. In a small mixing bowl, combine the lemon juice, mustard seeds, tarragon, pepper, garlic, and oil; mix well. 2. Place the chicken in a baking dish, and pour the marinade on top. Cover, and refrigerate overnight. 3. Grill the chicken over medium heat for 10–15 minutes, basting with the marinade. Serve hot.

Per Serving:

calorie: 239 | fat: 11g | protein: 28g | carbs: 8g | sugars: 2g | fiber: 2g | sodium: 54mg

Simply Terrific Turkey Meatballs

Prep time: 10 minutes | Cook time: 7 to 10 minutes |

Serves 4

1 red bell pepper, seeded and coarsely chopped	ground turkey
2 cloves garlic, coarsely chopped	1 egg, lightly beaten
¼ cup chopped fresh parsley	½ cup grated Parmesan cheese
1½ pounds (680 g) 85% lean	1 teaspoon salt
	½ teaspoon freshly ground black pepper

1. Preheat the air fryer to 400°F (204°C). 2. In a food processor fitted with a metal blade, combine the bell pepper, garlic, and parsley. Pulse until finely chopped. Transfer the vegetables to a large mixing bowl. 3. Add the turkey, egg, Parmesan, salt, and black pepper. Mix gently until thoroughly combined. Shape the mixture into 1¼-inch meatballs. 4. Working in batches if necessary, arrange the meatballs in a single layer in the air fryer basket; coat lightly with olive oil spray. Pausing halfway through the cooking time to shake the basket, air fry for 7 to 10 minutes, until lightly browned and a thermometer inserted into the center of a meatball registers 165°F (74°C).

Per Serving:

calories: 388 | fat: 25g | protein: 34g | carbs: 5g | fiber: 1g | sodium: 527mg

Turkey Stuffed Peppers

Prep time: 15 minutes | Cook time: 50 minutes |

Serves 4

1 teaspoon extra-virgin olive oil, plus more for greasing the baking dish
1 pound ground turkey breast
½ sweet onion, chopped
1 teaspoon minced garlic
1 tomato, diced

½ teaspoon chopped fresh basil
Sea salt
Freshly ground black pepper
4 red bell peppers, tops cut off, seeded
2 ounces low-sodium feta cheese

1. Preheat the oven to 350°F. 2. Lightly grease a 9-by-9-inch baking dish with olive oil and set it aside. 3. Place a large skillet over medium heat and add 1 teaspoon of olive oil. 4. Add the turkey to the skillet and cook until it is no longer pink, stirring occasionally to break up the meat and brown it evenly, about 6 minutes. 5. Add the onion and garlic and sauté until softened and translucent, about 3 minutes. 6. Stir in the tomato and basil. Season with salt and pepper. 7. Place the peppers cut-side up in the baking dish. Divide the filling into four equal portions and spoon it into the peppers. 8. Sprinkle the feta cheese on top of the filling. 9. Add ¼ cup of water to the dish and cover with aluminum foil. 10. Bake the peppers until they are soft and heated through, about 40 minutes.

Per Serving:

calorie: 285 | fat: 12g | protein: 31g | carbs: 12g | sugars: 8g | fiber: 3g | sodium: 79mg

Turkey Bolognese with Chickpea Pasta

Prep time: 5 minutes | Cook time: 25 minutes |

Serves 4

1 onion, coarsely chopped
1 large carrot, coarsely chopped
2 celery stalks, coarsely chopped
1 tablespoon extra-virgin olive oil
1 pound ground turkey

½ cup milk
¾ cup red or white wine
1 (28-ounce) can diced tomatoes
10 ounces cooked chickpea pasta

1. Place the onion, carrots, and celery in a food processor and pulse until finely chopped. 2. Heat the extra-virgin olive oil in a Dutch oven or medium skillet over medium-high heat. Sauté the chopped vegetables for 3 to 5 minutes, or until softened. Add the ground turkey, breaking the poultry into smaller pieces, and cook for 5 minutes. 3. Add the milk and wine and cook until the liquid is nearly evaporated (turn up the heat to high to quicken the process). 4. Add the tomatoes and bring the sauce to a simmer. Reduce the heat to low and simmer for 10 to 15 minutes. 5. Meanwhile, cook the pasta according to the package instructions and set aside. 6. Serve the sauce with the cooked chickpea pasta. 7. Store any leftovers in an airtight container in the refrigerator for 3 to 4 days.

Per Serving:

calorie: 419 | fat: 15g | protein: 31g | carbs: 34g | sugars: 8g | fiber: 11g | sodium: 150mg

Turkey Cabbage Soup

Prep time: 15 minutes | Cook time: 30 minutes |

Serves 4

1 tablespoon extra-virgin olive oil
1 sweet onion, chopped
2 celery stalks, chopped
2 teaspoons minced fresh garlic
4 cups finely shredded green cabbage
1 sweet potato, peeled, diced

8 cups chicken or turkey broth
2 bay leaves
1 cup chopped cooked turkey
2 teaspoons chopped fresh thyme
Sea salt
Freshly ground black pepper

1. Place a large saucepan over medium-high heat and add the olive oil. 2. Sauté the onion, celery, and garlic until softened and translucent, about 3 minutes. 3. Add the cabbage and sweet potato and sauté for 3 minutes. 4. Stir in the chicken broth and bay leaves and bring the soup to a boil. 5. Reduce the heat to low and simmer until the vegetables are tender, about 20 minutes. 6. Add the turkey and thyme and simmer until the turkey is heated through, about 4 minutes. 7. Remove the bay leaves and season the soup with salt and pepper.

Per Serving:

calorie: 444 | fat: 14g | protein: 38g | carbs: 46g | sugars: 17g | fiber: 7g | sodium: 427mg

Sesame-Ginger Chicken Soba

Prep time: 10 minutes | Cook time: 15 minutes |

Serves 6

8 ounces soba noodles
2 boneless, skinless chicken breasts, halved lengthwise
¼ cup tahini
2 tablespoons rice vinegar
1 tablespoon reduced-sodium gluten-free soy sauce or tamari
1 teaspoon toasted sesame oil

1 (1-inch) piece fresh ginger, finely grated
⅓ cup water
1 large cucumber, seeded and diced
1 scallions bunch, green parts only, cut into 1-inch segments
1 tablespoon sesame seeds

1. Preheat the broiler to high. 2. Bring a large pot of water to a boil. Add the noodles and cook until tender, according to the package directions. Drain and rinse the noodles in cool water. 3. On a baking sheet, arrange the chicken in a single layer. Broil for 5 to 7 minutes on each side, depending on the thickness, until the chicken is cooked through and its juices run clear. Use two forks to shred the chicken. 4. In a small bowl, combine the tahini, rice vinegar, soy sauce, sesame oil, ginger, and water. Whisk to combine. 5. In a large bowl, toss the shredded chicken, noodles, cucumber, and scallions. Pour the tahini sauce over the noodles and toss to combine. Served sprinkled with the sesame seeds.

Per Serving:

calories: 251 | fat: 8g | protein: 16g | carbs: 35g | sugars: 2g | fiber: 2g | sodium: 482mg

Tantalizing Jerked Chicken

Prep time: 10 minutes | Cook time: 20 minutes |
Serves 4

4 (5 ounces) boneless, skinless chicken breasts	1 tablespoon ground allspice
½ sweet onion, cut into chunks	2 teaspoons chopped fresh thyme
2 habanero chile peppers, halved lengthwise, seeded	1 teaspoon freshly ground black pepper
¼ cup freshly squeezed lime juice	½ teaspoon ground nutmeg
2 tablespoons extra-virgin olive oil	¼ teaspoon ground cinnamon
1 tablespoon minced garlic	2 cups fresh greens (such as arugula or spinach)
	1 cup halved cherry tomatoes

1. Place two chicken breasts in each of two large resealable plastic bags. Set them aside. 2. Place the onion, habaneros, lime juice, olive oil, garlic, allspice, thyme, black pepper, nutmeg, and cinnamon in a food processor and pulse until very well blended. 3. Pour half the marinade into each bag with the chicken breasts. Squeeze out as much air as possible, seal the bags, and place them in the refrigerator for 4 hours. 4. Preheat a barbecue to medium-high heat. 5. Let the chicken sit at room temperature for 15 minutes and then grill, turning at least once, until cooked through, about 15 minutes total. 6. Let the chicken rest for about 5 minutes before serving. Divide the greens and tomatoes among four serving plates, and top with the chicken.

Per Serving:

calorie: 268 | fat: 10g | protein: 33g | carbs: 9g | sugars: 4g | fiber: 2g | sodium: 74mg

Coconut Chicken Curry

Prep time: 15 minutes | Cook time: 35 minutes |
Serves 4

2 teaspoons extra-virgin olive oil	2 cups low-sodium chicken broth
3 (5 ounces) boneless, skinless chicken breasts, cut into 1-inch chunks	1 cup canned coconut milk
1 tablespoon grated fresh ginger	1 carrot, peeled and diced
1 tablespoon minced garlic	1 sweet potato, diced
2 tablespoons curry powder	2 tablespoons chopped fresh cilantro

1. Place a large saucepan over medium-high heat and add the oil. 2. Sauté the chicken until lightly browned and almost cooked through, about 10 minutes. 3. Add the ginger, garlic, and curry powder, and sauté until fragrant, about 3 minutes. 4. Stir in the chicken broth, coconut milk, carrot, and sweet potato and bring the mixture to a boil. 5. Reduce the heat to low and simmer, stirring occasionally, until the vegetables and chicken are tender, about 20 minutes. 6. Stir in the cilantro and serve.

Per Serving:

calorie: 327 | fat: 18g | protein: 29g | carbs: 14g | sugars: 2g | fiber: 3g | sodium: 122mg

Chicken with Lemon Caper Pan Sauce

Prep time: 10 minutes | Cook time: 15 minutes |
Serves 4

3 tablespoons extra-virgin olive oil	black pepper
4 chicken breast halves or thighs, pounded slightly to even thickness	¼ cup freshly squeezed lemon juice
	¼ cup dry white wine
½ teaspoon sea salt	2 tablespoons capers, rinsed
⅛ teaspoon freshly ground	2 tablespoons salted butter, very cold, cut into pieces

1. In a large skillet over medium-high heat, heat the olive oil until it shimmers. 2. Season the chicken with the salt and pepper. Add it to the hot oil and cook until opaque with an internal temperature of 165°F, about 5 minutes per side. Transfer the chicken to a plate and tent loosely with foil to keep warm. Keep the pan on the heat. 3. Add the lemon juice and wine to the pan, using the side of a spoon to scrape any browned bits from the bottom of the pan. Add the capers. Simmer until the liquid is reduced by half, about 3 minutes. Reduce the heat to low. 4. Whisk in the butter, one piece at a time, until incorporated. 5. Return the chicken to the pan, turning once to coat with the sauce. Serve with additional sauce spooned over the top.

Per Serving:

calorie: 367 | fat: 23g | protein: 37g | carbs: 2g | sugars: 1g | fiber: 0g | sodium: 591mg

Herbed Whole Turkey Breast

Prep time: 10 minutes | Cook time:30 minutes |
Serves 12

3 tablespoons extra-virgin olive oil	1 tablespoon kosher salt
1½ tablespoons herbes de Provence or poultry seasoning	1½ teaspoons freshly ground black pepper
2 teaspoons minced garlic	1 (6-pound) bone-in, skin-on whole turkey breast, rinsed and patted dry
1 teaspoon lemon zest (from 1 small lemon)	

1. In a small bowl, whisk together the olive oil, herbes de Provence, garlic, lemon zest, salt, and pepper. 2. Rub the outside of the turkey and under the skin with the olive oil mixture. 3. Pour 1 cup of water into the electric pressure cooker and insert a wire rack or trivet. 4. Place the turkey on the rack, skin-side up. 5. Close and lock the lid of the pressure cooker. Set the valve to sealing. 6. Cook on high pressure for 30 minutes. 7. When the cooking is complete, hit Cancel. Allow the pressure to release naturally for 20 minutes, then quick release any remaining pressure. 8. Once the pin drops, unlock and remove the lid. 9. Carefully transfer the turkey to a cutting board. Remove the skin, slice, and serve.

Per Serving:

calorie: 389 | fat: 19g | protein: 50g | carbs: 1g | sugars: 0g | fiber: 0g | sodium: 582mg

Buttermilk-Ginger Smothered Chicken

Prep time: 30 minutes | Cook time: 20 minutes | Serves 8

8 boneless, skinless chicken thighs
2 cups low-fat buttermilk
½ bunch fresh chives, thinly sliced
½ bunch fresh cilantro, thinly sliced
2 garlic cloves, minced
1 teaspoon ground ginger

1. Preheat the oven to 375°F. 2. In a large bowl, combine the chicken, buttermilk, chives, cilantro, garlic, and ginger, coating the chicken thoroughly. Cover and put in the refrigerator to marinate for at least 30 minutes. 3. Place the chicken in a Dutch oven and cover. Transfer to the oven and cook for 20 minutes, or until the chicken is moist on the inside and caramelized on the outside. 4. Serve.

Per Serving:

calorie: 363 | fat: 8g | protein: 64g | carbs: 4g | sugars: 3g | fiber: 0g | sodium: 188mg

Baked Chicken Stuffed with Collard Greens

Prep time: 10 minutes | Cook time: 30 minutes | Serves 4

For the gravy
2½ cups store-bought low-sodium chicken broth, divided
4 tablespoons whole-wheat flour, divided
1 medium yellow onion, chopped
½ bunch fresh thyme, roughly chopped
2 garlic cloves, minced
1 bay leaf
½ teaspoon celery seeds
1 teaspoon Worcestershire sauce
Freshly ground black pepper

For the chicken
2 boneless, skinless chicken breasts
Juice of 1 lime
1 teaspoon sweet paprika
½ teaspoon onion powder
½ teaspoon garlic powder
2 medium tomatoes, chopped
1 bunch collard greens, center stem removed, cut into 1-inch ribbons
¼ cup chicken broth (optional)
Generous pinch red pepper flakes

To make the gravy 1. In a shallow stockpot, combine ½ cup of broth and 1 tablespoon of flour and cook over medium-low heat, whisking until the flour is dissolved. Continue to add 1 cup of broth and the remaining 3 tablespoons of flour in increments until a thick sauce is formed. 2. Add the onion, thyme, garlic, bay leaf, and ½ cup of broth, stirring well. To make the chicken 1. Cut a slit in each chicken breast deep enough for stuffing along its entire length. 2. In a small mixing bowl, massage the chicken all over with the lime juice, paprika, onion powder, and garlic powder. 3. In an electric pressure cooker, combine the tomatoes and collard greens. If the mixture looks dry, add the chicken broth. 4. Close and lock the lid, and set the pressure valve to sealing. 5. Select the Manual/Pressure Cook setting, and cook for 2 minutes. 6. Once cooking is complete, quick-release the pressure. Carefully remove the lid. 7. Using tongs or a slotted spoon, remove the greens while leaving the tomatoes behind. 8. Stuff the chicken breasts with the greens. Lay on the bed of tomatoes in the pressure cooker, with the side with greens facing up. 9. Spoon half of the gravy over the stuffed chicken. 10. Close and lock the lid, and set the pressure valve to sealing. 11. Select the Manual/Pressure Cook setting, and cook for 10 minutes. 12. Once cooking is complete, quick-release the pressure. Carefully remove the lid. 13. Remove the chicken and tomatoes from pressure cooker, and transfer to a serving dish. Season with the red pepper flakes.

Per Serving:

calorie: 301 | fat: 6g | protein: 41g | carbs: 24g | sugars: 4g | fiber: 9g | sodium: 155mg

Unstuffed Peppers with Ground Turkey and Quinoa

Prep time: 0 minutes | Cook time: 35 minutes | Serves 8

2 tablespoons extra-virgin olive oil
1 yellow onion, diced
2 celery stalks, diced
2 garlic cloves, chopped
2 pounds 93 percent lean ground turkey
2 teaspoons Cajun seasoning blend (plus 1 teaspoon fine sea salt if using a salt-free blend)
½ teaspoon freshly ground black pepper
¼ teaspoon cayenne pepper
1 cup quinoa, rinsed
1 cup low-sodium chicken broth
One 14½ ounces can fire-roasted diced tomatoes and their liquid
3 red, orange, and/or yellow bell peppers, seeded and cut into 1-inch squares
1 green onion, white and green parts, thinly sliced
1½ tablespoons chopped fresh flat-leaf parsley
Hot sauce (such as Crystal or Frank's RedHot) for serving

1. Select the Sauté setting on the Instant Pot and heat the oil for 2 minutes. Add the onion, celery, and garlic and sauté for about 4 minutes, until the onion begins to soften. Add the turkey, Cajun seasoning, black pepper, and cayenne and sauté, using a wooden spoon or spatula to break up the meat as it cooks, for about 6 minutes, until cooked through and no streaks of pink remain. 2. Sprinkle the quinoa over the turkey in an even layer. Pour the broth and the diced tomatoes and their liquid over the quinoa, spreading the tomatoes on top. Sprinkle the bell peppers over the top in an even layer. 3. Secure the lid and set the Pressure Release to Sealing. Press the Cancel button to reset the cooking program, then select the Pressure Cook or Manual setting and set the cooking time for 8 minutes at high pressure. (The pot will take about 15 minutes to come up to pressure before the cooking program begins.) 4. When the cooking program ends, let the pressure release naturally for at least 15 minutes, then move the Pressure Release to Venting to release any remaining steam. Open the pot and sprinkle the green onion and parsley over the top in an even layer. 5. Spoon the unstuffed peppers into bowls, making sure to dig down to the bottom of the pot so each person gets an equal amount of peppers, quinoa, and meat. Serve hot, with hot sauce on the side.

Per Serving:

calories: 320 | fat: 14g | protein: 27g | carbs: 23g | sugars: 3g | fiber: 3g | sodium: 739mg

Tangy Barbecue Strawberry-Peach Chicken

Prep time: 20 minutes | Cook time: 40 minutes |

Serves 4

For the barbecue sauce
1 cup frozen peaches
1 cup frozen strawberries
¼ cup tomato purée
½ cup white vinegar
1 tablespoon yellow mustard
1 teaspoon mustard seeds
1 teaspoon turmeric
1 teaspoon sweet paprika

1 teaspoon garlic powder
½ teaspoon cayenne pepper
½ teaspoon onion powder
½ teaspoon freshly ground black pepper
1 teaspoon celery seeds
For the chicken
4 boneless, skinless chicken thighs

To make the barbecue sauce 1. In a stockpot, combine the peaches, strawberries, tomato purée, vinegar, mustard, mustard seeds, turmeric, paprika, garlic powder, cayenne, onion powder, black pepper, and celery seeds. Cook over low heat for 15 minutes, or until the flavors come together. 2. Remove the sauce from the heat, and let cool for 5 minutes. 3. Transfer the sauce to a blender, and purée until smooth. To make the chicken 1. Preheat the oven to 350°F. 2. Put the chicken in a medium bowl. Coat well with ½ cup of barbecue sauce. 3. Place the chicken on a rimmed baking sheet. 4. Place the baking sheet on the middle rack of the oven, and bake for about 20 minutes (depending on the thickness of thighs), or until the juices run clear. 5. Brush the chicken with additional sauce, return to the oven, and broil on high for 3 to 5 minutes, or until a light crust forms. 6. Serve.

Per Serving:

calorie: 389 | fat: 8g | protein: 63g | carbs: 13g | sugars: 7g | fiber: 3g | sodium: 175mg

Chicken Salad Salad

Prep time: 15 minutes | Cook time: 0 minutes |

Serves 4

2 cups shredded rotisserie chicken
1½ tablespoons plain low-fat Greek yogurt
⅛ teaspoon freshly ground black pepper

¼ cup halved purple seedless grapes
8 cups chopped romaine lettuce
1 medium tomato, sliced
1 avocado, sliced

1. In a large bowl, combine the chicken, yogurt, and pepper, and mix well. 2. Stir in the grapes. 3. Divide the lettuce into four portions. Spoon one-quarter of the chicken salad onto each portion and top with a couple slices of tomato and avocado.

Per Serving:

calorie: 305 | fat: 19g | protein: 24g | carbs: 11g | sugars: 4g | fiber: 6g | sodium: 79mg

Chicken with Mushroom Cream Sauce

Prep time: 5 minutes | Cook time: 20 minutes |

Serves 8

1 tablespoon extra-virgin olive oil
Eight 3-ounce boneless, skinless chicken breast halves
½ cup sliced mushrooms
3 tablespoons flour
½ cup low-sodium chicken

broth
¾ cup white wine
2 teaspoons lemon zest
½ teaspoons lemon pepper
1 cup plain fat-free Greek yogurt
Parsley sprigs

1. In a large nonstick skillet, heat the oil; add the chicken and cook for 5 minutes on each side. Remove the chicken, and keep warm. Add the mushrooms to the skillet, and cook until tender. 2. In a small bowl, whisk the flour with the broth and wine. Stir the mixture into the skillet, and add the lemon zest and pepper. Cook until thickened and bubbly. 3. Return the chicken to the skillet, and cook until the chicken is no longer pink. Transfer the chicken to a platter. Stir the yogurt into the skillet and heat thoroughly. Pour the sauce over the chicken, and garnish with parsley.

Per Serving:

calorie: 166 | fat: 4g | protein: 22g | carbs: 6g | sugars: 3g | fiber: 0g | sodium: 68mg

Herbed Cornish Hens

Prep time: 5 minutes | Cook time: 30 minutes |

Serves 8

4 Cornish hens, giblets removed (about 1¼ pound each)
2 cups white wine, divided
2 garlic cloves, minced
1 small onion, minced
½ teaspoon celery seeds

½ teaspoon poultry seasoning
½ teaspoon paprika
½ teaspoon dried oregano
¼ teaspoon freshly ground black pepper

1. Using a long, sharp knife, split each hen lengthwise. You may also buy precut hens. 2. Place the hens, cavity side up, on a rack in a shallow roasting pan. Pour 1½ cups of the wine over the hens; set aside. 3. In a shallow bowl, combine the garlic, onion, celery seeds, poultry seasoning, paprika, oregano, and pepper. Sprinkle half of the combined seasonings over the cavity of each split half. Cover, and refrigerate. Allow the hens to marinate for 2–3 hours. 4. Preheat the oven to 350 degrees. Bake the hens uncovered for 1 hour. Remove from the oven, turn breast side up, and remove the skin. Pour the remaining ½ cup of wine over the top, and sprinkle with the remaining seasonings. 5. Continue to bake for an additional 25–30 minutes, basting every 10 minutes until the hens are done. Transfer to a serving platter, and serve hot.

Per Serving:

calorie: 383 | fat: 10g | protein: 57g | carbs: 3g | sugars: 1g | fiber: 0g | sodium: 197mg

Speedy Chicken Cacciatore

Prep time: 5 minutes | Cook time: 30 minutes | Serves 6

2 pounds boneless, skinless chicken thighs
1½ teaspoons fine sea salt
½ teaspoon freshly ground black pepper
2 tablespoons extra-virgin olive oil
3 garlic cloves, chopped
2 large red bell peppers, seeded and cut into ¼ by 2-inch strips

2 large yellow onions, sliced
½ cup dry red wine
1½ teaspoons Italian seasoning
½ teaspoon red pepper flakes (optional)
One 14½-ounce can diced tomatoes and their liquid
2 tablespoons tomato paste
Cooked brown rice or whole-grain pasta for serving

1. Season the chicken thighs on both sides with 1 teaspoon of the salt and the black pepper. 2. Select the Sauté setting on the Instant Pot and heat the oil and garlic for 2 minutes, until the garlic is bubbling but not browned. Add the bell peppers, onions, and remaining ½ teaspoon salt and sauté for 3 minutes, until the onions begin to soften. Stir in the wine, Italian seasoning, and pepper flakes (if using). Using tongs, add the chicken to the pot, turning each piece to coat it in the wine and spices and nestling them in a single layer in the liquid. Pour the tomatoes and their liquid on top of the chicken and dollop the tomato paste on top. Do not stir them in. 3. Secure the lid and set the Pressure Release to Sealing. Press the Cancel button to reset the cooking program, then select the Poultry, Pressure Cook, or Manual setting and set the cooking time for 12 minutes at high pressure. (The pot will take about 15 minutes to come up to pressure before the cooking program begins.) 4. When the cooking program ends, perform a quick pressure release by moving the Pressure Release to Venting, or let the pressure release naturally. Open the pot and, using tongs, transfer the chicken and vegetables to a serving dish. 5. Spoon some of the sauce over the chicken and serve hot, with the rice on the side.

Per Serving:
calories: 297 | fat: 11g | protein: 32g | carbs: 16g | sugars: 3g | fiber: 3g | sodium: 772mg

Turkey Divan Casserole

Prep time: 10 minutes | Cook time: 50 minutes | Serves 6

Nonstick cooking spray
3 teaspoons extra-virgin olive oil, divided
1 pound turkey cutlets
Pinch salt
¼ teaspoon freshly ground black pepper, divided
¼ cup chopped onion
2 garlic cloves, minced
2 tablespoons whole-wheat

flour
1 cup unsweetened plain almond milk
1 cup low-sodium chicken broth
½ cup shredded Swiss cheese, divided
½ teaspoon dried thyme
4 cups chopped broccoli
¼ cup coarsely ground almonds

1. Preheat the oven to 375°F. Spray a baking dish with nonstick cooking spray. 2. In a skillet, heat 1 teaspoon of oil over medium heat. Season the turkey with the salt and ⅛ teaspoon of pepper. Sauté the turkey cutlets for 5 to 7 minutes on each side until cooked through. Transfer to a cutting board, cool briefly, and cut into bite-size pieces. 3. In the same pan, heat the remaining 2 teaspoons of oil over medium-high heat. Sauté the onion for 3 minutes until it begins to soften. Add the garlic and continue cooking for another minute. 4. Stir in the flour and mix well. Whisk in the almond milk, broth, and remaining ⅛ teaspoon of pepper, and continue whisking until smooth. Add ¼ cup of cheese and the thyme, and continue stirring until the cheese is melted. 5. In the prepared baking dish, arrange the broccoli on the bottom. Cover with half the sauce. Place the turkey pieces on top of the broccoli, and cover with the remaining sauce. Sprinkle with the remaining ¼ cup of cheese and the ground almonds. 6. Bake for 35 minutes until the sauce is bubbly and the top is browned.

Per Serving:
calories: 207 | fat: 8g | protein: 25g | carbs: 9g | sugars: 2g | fiber: 3g | sodium: 128mg

Roast Chicken with Pine Nuts and Fennel

Prep time: 20 minutes | Cook time: 30 minutes | Serves 2

For the herb paste
2 tablespoons fresh rosemary leaves
1 tablespoon freshly grated lemon zest
2 garlic cloves, quartered
½ teaspoon freshly ground black pepper
¼ teaspoon salt
1 teaspoon extra-virgin olive oil
For the chicken
4 (6 ounces) skinless chicken drumsticks

2 teaspoons extra-virgin olive oil
For the vegetables
1 large fennel bulb, cored and chopped (about 3 cups)
1 cup sliced fresh mushrooms
½ cup sliced carrots
¼ cup chopped sweet onion
2 teaspoons extra-virgin olive oil
2 tablespoons pine nuts
2 teaspoons white wine vinegar

To make the vegetables 1. Preheat the oven to 450°F. 2. In a 9-by-13-inch baking dish, toss together the fennel, mushrooms, carrots, onion, and olive oil. Place the dish in the preheated oven. Bake for 10 minutes. 3. Stir in the pine nuts. 4. Top with the browned drumsticks. Return the dish to the oven. Bake for 15 to 20 minutes more, or until the fennel is golden and an instant-read thermometer inserted into the thickest part of a drumstick without touching the bone registers 165°F. 5. Remove the chicken from the pan. 6. Stir the white wine vinegar into the pan. Toss the vegetables to coat, scraping up any browned bits. 7. Serve the chicken with the vegetables and enjoy!

Per Serving:
calorie: 316 | fat: 15g | protein: 35g | carbs: 10g | sugars: 4g | fiber: 3g | sodium: 384mg

Sautéed Chicken with Artichoke Hearts

Prep time: 5 minutes | Cook time: 20 minutes | Serves 4

Nonstick cooking spray
Three 8-ounce boneless,
skinless chicken breasts, halved
½ cup low-sodium chicken
stock
¼ cup dry white wine
Two 8 ounces cans artichoke
hearts, packed in water, drained
and quartered
1 medium onion, diced

1 medium green bell pepper,
chopped
2 tablespoons minced fresh
tarragon or mint
¼ teaspoon white pepper
2 teaspoons cornstarch
1 tablespoon cold water
2 medium tomatoes, cut into
wedges

1. Coat a large skillet with nonstick cooking spray; place over medium heat until hot. Add the chicken, and sauté until lightly browned, about 3–4 minutes per side. 2. Add the chicken stock, wine, artichokes, onion, green pepper, tarragon or mint, and white pepper; stir well. Bring to a boil, cover, reduce heat, and let simmer for 10–15 minutes or until the chicken is no longer pink and the vegetables are just tender. 3. In a small bowl, combine the cornstarch and water; add to the chicken mixture along with the tomato wedges, stirring until the mixture has thickened. Remove from the heat, and serve.

Per Serving:

calorie: 310 | fat: 5g | protein: 44g | carbs: 21g | sugars: 5g | fiber: 8g | sodium: 199mg

Asian Mushroom-Chicken Soup

Prep time: 30 minutes | Cook time: 15 minutes | Serves 6

1½ cups water
1 package (1 oz) dried
portabella or shiitake
mushrooms
1 tablespoon canola oil
¼ cup thinly sliced green
onions (4 medium)
2 tablespoons gingerroot,
peeled, minced
3 cloves garlic, minced
1 jalapeño chile, seeded,
minced
1 cup fresh snow pea pods,
sliced diagonally

3 cups reduced-sodium chicken
broth
1 can (8 ounces) sliced bamboo
shoots, drained
2 tablespoons low-sodium soy
sauce
½ teaspoon sriracha sauce
1 cup shredded cooked chicken
breast
1 cup cooked brown rice
4 teaspoons lime juice
½ cup thinly sliced fresh basil
leaves

1 In medium microwavable bowl, heat water uncovered on High 30 seconds or until hot. Add mushrooms; let stand 5 minutes or until tender. Drain mushrooms (reserve liquid). Slice any mushrooms that are large. Set aside. 2 In 4-quart saucepan, heat oil over medium heat. Add 2 tablespoons of the green onions, the gingerroot, garlic and chile to oil. Cook about 3 minutes, stirring occasionally, until vegetables are tender. Add snow pea pods; cook 2 minutes, stirring occasionally. Stir in mushrooms, reserved mushroom liquid and the remaining ingredients, except lime juice and basil. Heat to boiling;

reduce heat. Cover and simmer 10 minutes or until hot. Stir in lime juice. 3 Divide soup evenly among 6 bowls. Top servings with basil and remaining green onions.

Per Serving:

calories: 150 | fat: 4g | protein: 11g | carbs: 16g | sugars: 3g | fiber: 3g | sodium: 490mg

Wine-Poached Chicken with Herbs and Vegetables

Prep time: 5 minutes | Cook time: 1 hour | Serves 8

4 quarts low-sodium chicken
broth
2 cups dry white wine
4 large bay leaves
4 sprigs fresh thyme
¼ teaspoon freshly ground
black pepper
4 pounds chicken, giblets
removed, washed and patted

dry
½ pound carrots, peeled and
julienned
½ pound turnips, peeled and
julienned
½ pound parsnips, peeled and
julienned
4 small leeks, washed and
trimmed

1. In a large stockpot, combine the broth, wine, bay leaves, thyme, dash salt (optional), and pepper. Let simmer over medium heat while you prepare the chicken. 2. Stuff the cavity with ⅓ each of the carrots, turnips, and parsnips; then truss. Add the stuffed chicken to the stockpot, and poach, covered, over low heat for 30 minutes. 3. Add the remaining vegetables with the leeks, and continue to simmer for 25–30 minutes, or until juices run clear when the chicken is pierced with a fork. 4. Remove the chicken and vegetables to a serving platter. Carve the chicken, remove the skin, and surround the sliced meat with poached vegetables to serve.

Per Serving:

calorie: 476 | fat: 13g | protein: 57g | carbs: 24g | sugars: 6g | fiber: 4g | sodium: 387mg

Lemon-Basil Turkey Breasts

Prep time: 30 minutes | Cook time: 58 minutes | Serves 4

2 tablespoons olive oil
2 pounds (907 g) turkey breasts,
bone-in, skin-on
Coarse sea salt and ground
black pepper, to taste

1 teaspoon fresh basil leaves,
chopped
2 tablespoons lemon zest,
grated

1. Rub olive oil on all sides of the turkey breasts; sprinkle with salt, pepper, basil, and lemon zest. 2. Place the turkey breasts skin side up on the parchment-lined air fryer basket. 3. Cook in the preheated air fryer at 330ºF (166ºC) for 30 minutes. Now, turn them over and cook an additional 28 minutes. 4. Serve with lemon wedges, if desired. Bon appétit!

Per Serving:

calories: 417 | fat: 23g | protein: 50g | carbs: 0g | fiber: 0g | sodium: 134mg

One-Pan Chicken Dinner

**Prep time: 5 minutes | Cook time: 35 minutes |
Serves 4**

3 tablespoons extra-virgin olive oil
1 tablespoon red wine vinegar or apple cider vinegar
¼ teaspoon garlic powder
3 tablespoons Italian seasoning

4 (4ounces) boneless, skinless chicken breasts
2 cups cubed sweet potatoes
20 Brussels sprouts, halved lengthwise

1. Preheat the oven to 400ºF. 2. In a large bowl, whisk together the oil, vinegar, garlic powder, and Italian seasoning. 3. Add the chicken, sweet potatoes, and Brussels sprouts, and coat thoroughly with the marinade. 4. Remove the ingredients from the marinade and arrange them on a baking sheet in a single layer. Roast for 15 minutes. 5. Remove the baking sheet from the oven, flip the chicken over, and bake for another 15 to 20 minutes.

Per Serving:
calorie: 346 | fat: 13g | protein: 30g | carbs: 26g | sugars: 6g | fiber: 7g | sodium: 575mg

Pulled BBQ Chicken and Texas-Style Cabbage Slaw

**Prep time: 5 minutes | Cook time: 20 minutes |
Serves 6**

Chicken
1 cup water
¼ teaspoon fine sea salt
3 garlic cloves, peeled
2 bay leaves
2 pounds boneless, skinless chicken thighs (see Note)
Cabbage Slaw
½ head red or green cabbage, thinly sliced
1 red bell pepper, seeded and thinly sliced
2 jalapeño chiles, seeded and

cut into narrow strips
2 carrots, julienned
1 large Fuji or Gala apple, julienned
½ cup chopped fresh cilantro
3 tablespoons fresh lime juice
3 tablespoons extra-virgin olive oil
½ teaspoon ground cumin
¼ teaspoon fine sea salt
¾ cup low-sugar or unsweetened barbecue sauce
Cornbread, for serving

1. To make the chicken: Combine the water, salt, garlic, bay leaves, and chicken thighs in the Instant Pot, arranging the chicken in a single layer. 2. Secure the lid and set the Pressure Release to Sealing. Select the Poultry, Pressure Cook, or Manual setting and set the cooking time for 10 minutes at high pressure. (The pot will take about 10 minutes to come up to pressure before the cooking program begins.) 3. To make the slaw: While the chicken is cooking, in a large bowl, combine the cabbage, bell pepper, jalapeños, carrots, apple, cilantro, lime juice, oil, cumin, and salt and toss together until the vegetables and apples are evenly coated. 4. When the cooking program ends, perform a quick pressure release by moving the Pressure Release to Venting, or let the pressure release naturally. Open the pot and, using tongs, transfer the chicken to a cutting board. Using two forks, shred the chicken

into bite-size pieces. Wearing heat-resistant mitts, lift out the inner pot and discard the cooking liquid. Return the inner pot to the housing. 5. Return the chicken to the pot and stir in the barbecue sauce. You can serve it right away or heat it for a minute or two on the Sauté setting, then return the pot to its Keep Warm setting until ready to serve. 6. Divide the chicken and slaw evenly among six plates. Serve with wedges of cornbread on the side.

Per Serving:
calories: 320 | fat: 14g | protein: 32g | carbs: 18g | sugars: 7g | fiber: 4g | sodium: 386mg

Ann's Chicken Cacciatore

**Prep time: 25 minutes | Cook time: 3 to 9 minutes |
Serves 8**

1 large onion, thinly sliced
3 pound chicken, cut up, skin removed, trimmed of fat
2 6 ounces cans tomato paste
4 ounces can sliced mushrooms, drained
1 teaspoon salt
¼ cup dry white wine

¼ teaspoons pepper
1 to 2 garlic cloves, minced
1 to 2 teaspoons dried oregano
½ teaspoon dried basil
½ teaspoon celery seed, optional
1 bay leaf

1. In the inner pot of the Instant Pot, place the onion and chicken. 2. Combine remaining ingredients and pour over the chicken. 3. Secure the lid and make sure vent is at sealing. Cook on Slow Cook mode, low 7 to 9 hours, or high 3 to 4 hours.

Per Serving:
calories: 161 | fat: 4g | protein: 19g | carbs: 12g | sugars: 3g | fiber: 3g | sodium: 405mg

Wild Rice and Turkey Casserole

**Prep time: 10 minutes | Cook time: 55 minutes |
Serves 6**

2 cups cut-up cooked turkey or chicken
2¼ cups boiling water
⅓ cup fat-free (skim) milk
4 medium green onions, sliced (¼ cup)
1 can (10.75 ounces) condensed

98% fat-free cream of mushroom soup
1 package (6 ounces) original long-grain and wild rice mix
Additional green onions, if desired

1. Heat oven to 350°F. In ungreased 2-quart casserole, mix all ingredients, including seasoning packet from rice mix. 2. Cover; bake 45 to 50 minutes or until rice is tender. Uncover; bake 10 to 15 minutes longer or until liquid is absorbed. Sprinkle with additional green onions.

Per Serving:
calories: 220 | fat: 5g | protein: 17g | carbs: 27g | sugars: 2g | fiber: 1g | sodium: 740mg

Jerk Chicken Thighs

Prep time: 30 minutes | Cook time: 15 to 20 minutes | Serves 6

2 teaspoons ground coriander
1 teaspoon ground allspice
1 teaspoon cayenne pepper
1 teaspoon ground ginger
1 teaspoon salt
1 teaspoon dried thyme
½ teaspoon ground cinnamon
½ teaspoon ground nutmeg
2 pounds (907 g) boneless chicken thighs, skin on
2 tablespoons olive oil

1. In a small bowl, combine the coriander, allspice, cayenne, ginger, salt, thyme, cinnamon, and nutmeg. Stir until thoroughly combined. 2. Place the chicken in a baking dish and use paper towels to pat dry. Thoroughly coat both sides of the chicken with the spice mixture. Cover and refrigerate for at least 2 hours, preferably overnight. 3. Preheat the air fryer to 360°F (182°C). 4. Working in batches if necessary, arrange the chicken in a single layer in the air fryer basket and lightly coat with the olive oil. Pausing halfway through the cooking time to flip the chicken, air fry for 15 to 20 minutes, until a thermometer inserted into the thickest part registers 165°F (74°C).

Per Serving:

calories: 227 | fat: 11g | protein: 30g | carbs: 1g | fiber: 0g | sodium: 532mg

Peppered Chicken with Balsamic Kale

Prep time: 5 minutes | Cook time: 15 minutes | Serves 4

4 (4 ounces) boneless, skinless chicken breasts
¼ teaspoon salt
1 tablespoon freshly ground black pepper
2 tablespoons unsalted butter
1 tablespoon extra-virgin olive
oil
8 cups stemmed and roughly chopped kale, loosely packed (about 2 bunches)
½ cup balsamic vinegar
20 cherry tomatoes, halved

1. Season both sides of the chicken breasts with the salt and pepper. 2. Heat a large skillet over medium heat. When hot, heat the butter and oil. Add the chicken and cook for 8 to 10 minutes, flipping halfway through. When cooked all the way through, remove the chicken from the skillet and set aside. 3. Increase the heat to medium-high. Put the kale in the skillet and cook for 3 minutes, stirring every minute. 4. Add the vinegar and the tomatoes and cook for another 3 to 5 minutes. 5. Divide the kale and tomato mixture into four equal portions, and top each portion with 1 chicken breast.

Per Serving:

calorie: 383 | fat: 12g | protein: 34g | carbs: 38g | sugars: 25g | fiber: 11g | sodium: 256mg

Creamy Nutmeg Chicken

Prep time: 20 minutes | Cook time: 10 minutes | Serves 6

1 tablespoon canola oil
6 boneless chicken breast halves, skin and visible fat removed
¼ cup chopped onion
¼ cup minced parsley
2 (10¾-ounce) cans 98% fat-free, reduced-sodium cream of
mushroom soup
½ cup fat-free sour cream
½ cup fat-free milk
1 tablespoon ground nutmeg
¼ teaspoon sage
¼ teaspoon dried thyme
¼ teaspoon crushed rosemary

1. Press the Sauté button on the Instant Pot and then add the canola oil. Place the chicken in the oil and brown chicken on both sides. Remove the chicken to a plate. 2. Sauté the onion and parsley in the remaining oil in the Instant Pot until the onions are tender. Press Cancel on the Instant Pot, then place the chicken back inside. 3. Mix together the remaining ingredients in a bowl then pour over the chicken. 4. Secure the lid and set the vent to sealing. Set on Manual mode for 10 minutes. 5. When cooking time is up, let the pressure release naturally.

Per Serving:

calories: 264 | fat: 8g | protein: 31g | carbs: 15g | sugars: 5g | fiber: 1g | sodium: 495mg

Chicken Patties

Prep time: 15 minutes | Cook time: 12 minutes | Serves 4

1 pound (454 g) ground chicken thigh meat
½ cup shredded Mozzarella cheese
1 teaspoon dried parsley
½ teaspoon garlic powder
¼ teaspoon onion powder
1 large egg
2 ounces (57 g) pork rinds, finely ground

1. In a large bowl, mix ground chicken, Mozzarella, parsley, garlic powder, and onion powder. Form into four patties. 2. Place patties in the freezer for 15 to 20 minutes until they begin to firm up. 3. Whisk egg in a medium bowl. Place the ground pork rinds into a large bowl. 4. Dip each chicken patty into the egg and then press into pork rinds to fully coat. Place patties into the air fryer basket. 5. Adjust the temperature to 360°F (182°C) and air fry for 12 minutes. 6. Patties will be firm and cooked to an internal temperature of 165°F (74°C) when done. Serve immediately.

Per Serving:

calories: 265 | fat: 15g | protein: 29g | carbs: 1g | fiber: 0g | sodium: 285mg

Baked Turkey Spaghetti

Prep time: 5 minutes | Cook time: 20 minutes |
Serves 4

1 (10 ounces) package zucchini noodles
2 tablespoons extra-virgin olive oil, divided
1 pound 93% lean ground turkey

½ teaspoon dried oregano
2 cups low-sodium spaghetti sauce
½ cup shredded sharp Cheddar cheese

1. Pat zucchini noodles dry between two paper towels. 2. In an oven-safe medium skillet, heat 1 tablespoon of olive oil over medium heat. When hot, add the zucchini noodles. Cook for 3 minutes, stirring halfway through. 3. Add the remaining 1 tablespoon of oil, ground turkey, and oregano. Cook for 7 to 10 minutes, stirring and breaking apart, as needed. 4. Add the spaghetti sauce to the skillet and stir. 5. If your broiler is in the top of your oven, place the oven rack in the center position. Set the broiler on high. 6. Top the mixture with the cheese, and broil for 5 minutes or until the cheese is bubbly.

Per Serving:

calorie: 365 | fat: 23g | protein: 27g | carbs: 13g | sugars: 9g | fiber: 3g | sodium: 214mg

Coconut Lime Chicken

Prep time: 5 minutes | Cook time: 15 minutes |
Serves 4

1 tablespoon coconut oil
4 (4 ounces) boneless, skinless chicken breasts
½ teaspoon salt
1 red bell pepper, cut into ¼-inch-thick slices
16 asparagus spears, bottom ends trimmed

1 cup unsweetened coconut milk
2 tablespoons freshly squeezed lime juice
½ teaspoon garlic powder
¼ teaspoon red pepper flakes
¼ cup chopped fresh cilantro

1. In a large skillet, heat the oil over medium-low heat. When hot, add the chicken. 2. Season the chicken with the salt. Cook for 5 minutes, then flip. 3. Push the chicken to the side of the skillet, and add the bell pepper and asparagus. Cook, covered, for 5 minutes. 4. Meanwhile, in a small bowl, whisk together the coconut milk, lime juice, garlic powder, and red pepper flakes. 5. Add the coconut milk mixture to the skillet, and boil over high heat for 2 to 3 minutes. 6. Top with the cilantro.

Per Serving:

calorie: 319 | fat: 21g | protein: 28g | carbs: 7g | sugars: 4g | fiber: 2g | sodium: 353mg

Chicken Satay Stir-Fry

Prep time: 10 minutes | Cook time: 15 minutes |
Serves 4

3 tablespoons extra-virgin olive oil
1 pound chicken breasts or thighs, cut into ¾-inch pieces
½ teaspoon sea salt
2 cups broccoli florets
1 red bell pepper, seeded and

chopped
6 scallions, green and white parts, sliced on the bias (cut diagonally into thin slices)
1 head cauliflower, riced
Peanut Sauce

1. In a large skillet over medium-high heat, heat the olive oil until it shimmers. 2. Season the chicken with the salt. Add the chicken to the oil and cook, stirring occasionally, until opaque, about 5 minutes. Remove the chicken from the oil with a slotted spoon and set it aside on a plate. Return the pan to the heat. 3. Add the broccoli, bell pepper, and scallions. Cook, stirring, until the vegetables are crisp-tender, 3 to 5 minutes. Add the cauliflower and cook for 3 minutes more. 4. Return the chicken to the skillet. Stir in the Peanut Sauce. Bring to a simmer and reduce heat to medium-low. Simmer to heat through, about 2 minutes more.

Per Serving:

calorie: 283 | fat: 15g | protein: 26g | carbs: 11g | sugars: 4g | fiber: 4g | sodium: 453mg

Easy Chicken Cacciatore

Prep time: 5 minutes | Cook time: 20 minutes |
Serves 2

Extra-virgin olive oil cooking spray
1 garlic clove, chopped
½ cup chopped red onion
¾ cup chopped green bell pepper
2 (6 ounces) boneless skinless

chicken breasts, cubed
1 cup sliced cremini mushrooms
½ cup chopped tomatoes, with juice
1 cup green beans
1 teaspoon dried oregano
1 teaspoon dried rosemary

1. Coat a skillet with cooking spray. Place it over medium heat. 2. Add the garlic. Sauté for about 1 minute, or until browned. 3. Add the red onion, green bell pepper, and chicken. Cook for about 6 minutes, or until the chicken is slightly browned, tossing to cook all sides. 4. Stir in the mushrooms, tomatoes, green beans, oregano, and rosemary. Reduce the heat to medium-low. Simmer for 8 to 10 minutes, stirring constantly. 5. Remove from the heat and serve hot. 6. Enjoy!

Per Serving:

calorie: 265 | fat: 5g | protein: 42g | carbs: 13g | sugars: 6g | fiber: 4g | sodium: 91mg

Spice-Rubbed Chicken Thighs

Prep time: 10 minutes | Cook time: 25 minutes | Serves 4

4 (4 ounces / 113 g) bone-in, skin-on chicken thighs
½ teaspoon salt
½ teaspoon garlic powder
2 teaspoons chili powder

1 teaspoon paprika
1 teaspoon ground cumin
1 small lime, halved

1. Pat chicken thighs dry and sprinkle with salt, garlic powder, chili powder, paprika, and cumin. 2. Squeeze juice from ½ lime over thighs. Place thighs into ungreased air fryer basket. Adjust the temperature to 380°F (193°C) and roast for 25 minutes, turning thighs halfway through cooking. Thighs will be crispy and browned with an internal temperature of at least 165°F (74°C) when done. 3. Transfer thighs to a large serving plate and drizzle with remaining lime juice. Serve warm.

Per Serving:

calories: 151 | fat: 5g | protein: 23g | carbs: 3g | fiber: 1g | sodium: 439mg

Chicken Provençal

Prep time: 5 minutes | Cook time: 25 minutes | Serves 4

2 tablespoons extra-virgin olive oil
Two 8-ounce boneless, skinless chicken breasts, halved
1 medium garlic clove, minced
¼ cup minced onion
¼ cup minced green bell pepper

½ cup dry white wine
1 cup canned diced tomatoes
¼ cup pitted Kalamata olives
¼ cup finely chopped fresh basil
⅛ teaspoon freshly ground black pepper

1. Heat the oil in a skillet over medium heat. Add the chicken, and brown about 3–5 minutes. 2. Add the remaining ingredients, and cook uncovered over medium heat for 20 minutes or until the chicken is no longer pink. Transfer to a serving platter and season with additional pepper to taste, if desired, before serving.

Per Serving:

calorie: 245 | fat: 11g | protein: 26g | carbs: 5g | sugars: 2g | fiber: 2g | sodium: 121mg

Chapter 6 Fish and Seafood

Broiled Sole with Mustard Sauce

Prep time: 5 minutes | Cook time: 20 minutes |
Serves 6

Nonstick cooking spray
1½ pound fresh sole filets
3 tablespoons low-fat mayonnaise
2 tablespoons Dijon mustard
2 tablespoons chopped parsley
⅛ teaspoon freshly ground black pepper
1 large lemon, cut into wedges

1. Preheat broiler. Coat a baking sheet with nonstick cooking spray. Arrange the filets so they don't overlap. 2. In a small bowl, combine the mayonnaise, mustard, parsley, and pepper, and mix thoroughly. Spread the mixture evenly over the filets. Broil 3–4 inches from the heat for 4 minutes until the fish flakes easily with a fork. 3. Arrange the filets on a serving platter, garnish with lemon wedges, and serve.

Per Serving:

calories: 104 | fat: 4g | protein: 14g | carbs: 3g | sugars: 1g | fiber: 1g | sodium: 402mg

Shrimp Étouffée

Prep time: 20 minutes | Cook time: 30 minutes |
Serves 4 to 6

2 cups store-bought low-sodium vegetable broth, divided
¼ cup whole-wheat flour
1 small onion, finely chopped
2 celery stalks including leaves, finely chopped
1 medium green bell pepper, finely chopped
1 medium poblano pepper, finely chopped
3 garlic cloves, minced
1 tablespoon Creole seasoning
2 pounds medium shrimp, shelled and deveined
⅓ cup finely chopped chives, for garnish

1. In a Dutch oven, bring ½ cup of broth to a simmer over medium heat. 2. Stir in the flour and reduce the heat to low. Cook, stirring often, for 5 minutes, or until a thick paste is formed. 3. Add ½ cup of broth, the onion, celery, bell pepper, poblano pepper, and garlic and cook for 2 to 5 minutes, or until the vegetables have softened. 4. Slowly add the seasoning and remaining 1 cup of broth, ¼ cup at a time. 5. Add the shrimp and cook for about 5 minutes, or until just opaque. 6. Serve with the vegetable of your choice. Garnish with the chives.

Per Serving:

calories: 164 | fat: 1g | protein: 32g | carbs: 8g | sugars: 2g | fiber: 1g | sodium: 500mg

Tuna Steaks with Olive Tapenade

Prep time: 10 minutes | Cook time: 10 minutes |
Serves 4

4 (6 ounces / 170 g) ahi tuna steaks
1 tablespoon olive oil
Salt and freshly ground black pepper, to taste
½ lemon, sliced into 4 wedges
Olive Tapenade:
½ cup pitted kalamata olives
1 tablespoon olive oil
1 tablespoon chopped fresh parsley
1 clove garlic
2 teaspoons red wine vinegar
1 teaspoon capers, drained

1. Preheat the air fryer to 400°F (204°C). 2. Drizzle the tuna steaks with the olive oil and sprinkle with salt and black pepper. Arrange the tuna steaks in a single layer in the air fryer basket. Pausing to turn the steaks halfway through the cooking time, air fry for 10 minutes until the fish is firm. 3. To make the tapenade: In a food processor fitted with a metal blade, combine the olives, olive oil, parsley, garlic, vinegar, and capers. Pulse until the mixture is finely chopped, pausing to scrape down the sides of the bowl if necessary. Spoon the tapenade over the top of the tuna steaks and serve with lemon wedges.

Per Serving:

calories: 269 | fat: 9g | protein: 42g | carbs: 2g | fiber: 1g | sodium: 252mg

Grilled Rosemary Swordfish

Prep time: 5 minutes | Cook time: 15 minutes |
Serves 4

2 scallions, thinly sliced
2 tablespoons extra-virgin olive oil
2 tablespoons white wine vinegar
1 teaspoon fresh rosemary, finely chopped
4 swordfish steaks (1 pound total)

1. In a small bowl, combine the scallions, olive oil, vinegar, and rosemary. Pour over the swordfish steaks. Let the steaks marinate for 30 minutes. 2. Remove the steaks from the marinade, and grill for 5–7 minutes per side, brushing with marinade. Transfer to a serving platter, and serve.

Per Serving:

calories: 225 | fat: 14g | protein: 22g | carbs: 0g | sugars: 0g | fiber: 0g | sodium: 92mg

Ceviche

Prep time: 10 minutes | Cook time: 0 minutes |

Serves 4

½ pound fresh skinless, white, ocean fish fillet (halibut, mahi mahi, etc.), diced
1 cup freshly squeezed lime juice, divided
2 tablespoons chopped fresh cilantro, divided
1 serrano pepper, sliced

1 garlic clove, crushed
¾ teaspoon salt, divided
½ red onion, thinly sliced
2 tomatoes, diced
1 red bell pepper, seeded and diced
1 tablespoon extra-virgin olive oil

1. In a large mixing bowl, combine the fish, ¾ cup of lime juice, 1 tablespoon of cilantro, serrano pepper, garlic, and ½ teaspoon of salt. The fish should be covered or nearly covered in lime juice. Cover the bowl and refrigerate for 4 hours. 2. Sprinkle the remaining ¼ teaspoon of salt over the onion in a small bowl, and let sit for 10 minutes. Drain and rinse well. 3. In a large bowl, combine the tomatoes, bell pepper, olive oil, remaining ¼ cup of lime juice, and onion. Let rest for at least 10 minutes, or as long as 4 hours, while the fish "cooks." 4. When the fish is ready, it will be completely white and opaque. At this time, strain the juice, reserving it in another bowl. If desired, remove the serrano pepper and garlic. 5. Add the vegetables to the fish, and stir gently. Taste, and add some of the reserved lime juice to the ceviche as desired. Serve topped with the remaining 1 tablespoon of cilantro.

Per Serving:

calories: 121 | fat: 4g | protein: 12g | carbs: 11g | sugars: 5g | fiber: 2g | sodium: 405mg

Cucumber and Salmon Salad

Prep time: 10 minutes | Cook time: 8 to 10 minutes |

Serves 2

1 pound (454 g) salmon fillet
1½ tablespoons olive oil, divided
1 tablespoon sherry vinegar
1 tablespoon capers, rinsed and drained
1 seedless cucumber, thinly

sliced
¼ Vidalia onion, thinly sliced
2 tablespoons chopped fresh parsley
Salt and freshly ground black pepper, to taste

1. Preheat the air fryer to 400°F (204°C). 2. Lightly coat the salmon with ½ tablespoon of the olive oil. Place skin-side down in the air fryer basket and air fry for 8 to 10 minutes until the fish is opaque and flakes easily with a fork. Transfer the salmon to a plate and let cool to room temperature. Remove the skin and carefully flake the fish into bite-size chunks. 3. In a small bowl, whisk the remaining 1 tablespoon olive oil and the vinegar until thoroughly combined. Add the flaked fish, capers, cucumber, onion, and parsley. Season to taste with salt and freshly ground black pepper. Toss gently to coat. Serve immediately or cover and refrigerate for up to 4 hours.

Per Serving:

calories: 399 | fat: 20g | protein: 47g | carbs: 4g | fiber: 1g | sodium: 276mg

Seafood Stew

Prep time: 20 minutes | Cook time: 30 minutes |

Serves 6

1 tablespoon extra-virgin olive oil
1 sweet onion, chopped
2 teaspoons minced garlic
3 celery stalks, chopped
2 carrots, peeled and chopped
1 (28 ounces) can sodium-free diced tomatoes, undrained
3 cups low-sodium chicken broth
½ cup clam juice
¼ cup dry white wine
2 teaspoons chopped fresh basil

2 teaspoons chopped fresh oregano
2 (4 ounces) haddock fillets, cut into 1-inch chunks
1 pound mussels, scrubbed, debearded
8 ounces (16–20 count) shrimp, peeled, deveined, quartered
Sea salt
Freshly ground black pepper
2 tablespoons chopped fresh parsley

1. Place a large saucepan over medium-high heat and add the olive oil. 2. Sauté the onion and garlic until softened and translucent, about 3 minutes. 3. Stir in the celery and carrots and sauté for 4 minutes. 4. Stir in the tomatoes, chicken broth, clam juice, white wine, basil, and oregano. 5. Bring the sauce to a boil, then reduce the heat to low. Simmer for 15 minutes. 6. Add the fish and mussels, cover, and cook until the mussels open, about 5 minutes. 7. Discard any unopened mussels. Add the shrimp to the pan and cook until the shrimp are opaque, about 2 minutes. 8. Season with salt and pepper. Serve garnished with the chopped parsley.

Per Serving:

calories: 230 | fat: 6g | protein: 27g | carbs: 18g | sugars: 8g | fiber: 4g | sodium: 490mg

Faux Conch Fritters

Prep time: 15 minutes | Cook time: 20 minutes |

Serves 4

4 medium egg whites
½ cup fat-free milk
1 cup chickpea crumbs
¼ teaspoon freshly ground black pepper
½ teaspoon ground cumin
3 cups frozen chopped scallops,

thawed
1 small onion, finely chopped
1 small green bell pepper, finely chopped
2 celery stalks, finely chopped
2 garlic cloves, minced
Juice of 2 limes

1. Preheat the oven to 350°F. 2. In a large bowl, combine the egg whites, milk, and chickpea crumbs. 3. Add the black pepper and cumin and mix well. 4. Add the scallops, onion, bell pepper, celery, and garlic. 5. Form golf ball–size patties and place on a rimmed baking sheet 1 inch apart. 6. Transfer the baking sheet to the oven and cook for 5 to 7 minutes, or until golden brown. 7. Flip the patties, return to the oven, and bake for 5 to 7 minutes, or until golden brown. 8. Top with the lime juice, and serve.

Per Serving:

calories: 280 | fat: 4g | protein: 23g | carbs: 40g | sugars: 9g | fiber: 7g | sodium: 327mg

Scallops and Asparagus Skillet

Prep time: 10 minutes | Cook time: 15 minutes |

Serves 4

3 teaspoons extra-virgin olive oil, divided
1 pound asparagus, trimmed and cut into 2-inch segments
1 tablespoon butter
1 pound sea scallops

¼ cup dry white wine
Juice of 1 lemon
2 garlic cloves, minced
¼ teaspoon freshly ground black pepper

1. In a large skillet, heat 1½ teaspoons of oil over medium heat. 2. Add the asparagus and sauté for 5 to 6 minutes until just tender, stirring regularly. Remove from the skillet and cover with aluminum foil to keep warm. 3. Add the remaining 1½ teaspoons of oil and the butter to the skillet. When the butter is melted and sizzling, place the scallops in a single layer in the skillet. Cook for about 3 minutes on one side until nicely browned. Use tongs to gently loosen and flip the scallops, and cook on the other side for another 3 minutes until browned and cooked through. Remove and cover with foil to keep warm. 4. In the same skillet, combine the wine, lemon juice, garlic, and pepper. Bring to a simmer for 1 to 2 minutes, stirring to mix in any browned pieces left in the pan. 5. Return the asparagus and the cooked scallops to the skillet to coat with the sauce. Serve warm.

Per Serving:
calories: 252 | fat: 7g | protein: 26g | carbs: 15g | sugars: 3g | fiber: 2g | sodium: 493mg

Grilled Scallop Kabobs

Prep time: 15 minutes | Cook time: 20 minutes |

Serves 6

15 ounces pineapple chunks, packed in their own juice, undrained
¼ cup dry white wine
¼ cup light soy sauce
2 tablespoons minced fresh parsley
4 garlic cloves, minced

⅛ teaspoon freshly ground black pepper
1 pound scallops
18 large cherry tomatoes
1 large green bell pepper, cut into 1-inch squares
18 medium mushroom caps

1. Drain the pineapple, reserving the juice. In a shallow baking dish, combine the pineapple juice, wine, soy sauce, parsley, garlic, and pepper. Mix well. 2. Add the pineapple, scallops, tomatoes, green pepper, and mushrooms to the marinade. Marinate 30 minutes at room temperature, stirring occasionally. 3. Alternate pineapple, scallops, and vegetables on metal or wooden skewers (remember to soak wooden skewers in water before using). 4. Grill the kabobs over medium-hot coals about 4–5 inches from the heat, turning frequently, for 5–7 minutes.

Per Serving:
calories: 132 | fat: 1g | protein: 13g | carbs: 18g | sugars: 10g | fiber: 3g | sodium: 587mg

Fish Tacos

Prep time: 5 minutes | Cook time: 10 minutes |

Serves 4

For the Tacos
2 tablespoons extra-virgin olive oil
4 (6 ounces) cod fillets
8 (10-inch) yellow corn tortillas
2 cups packaged shredded cabbage
¼ cup chopped fresh cilantro

4 lime wedges
For the Sauce
½ cup plain low-fat Greek yogurt
⅓ cup low-fat mayonnaise
½ teaspoon garlic powder
½ teaspoon ground cumin

To Make the Tacos 1. Heat a medium skillet over medium-low heat. When hot, pour the oil into the skillet, then add the fish and cover. Cook for 4 minutes, then flip and cook for 4 minutes more. 2. Top each tortilla with one-eighth of the cabbage, sauce, cilantro, and fish. Finish each taco with a squeeze of lime. To Make the Sauce 3. In a small bowl, whisk together the yogurt, mayonnaise, garlic powder, and cumin.

Per Serving:
calories: 373 | fat: 13g | protein: 36g | carbs: 30g | sugars: 4g | fiber: 4g | sodium: 342mg

Lemon-Pepper Salmon with Roasted Broccoli

Prep time: 5 minutes | Cook time: 20 minutes |

Serves 4

4 (6 ounces [170 g]) salmon fillets
Cooking oil spray, as needed
Juice of 1 medium lemon (see Tips)
½ teaspoon black pepper

¼ teaspoon garlic salt or ¼ teaspoon sea salt mixed with ¼ teaspoon garlic powder
1 pound (454 g) broccoli florets
¼ teaspoon sea salt
¼ teaspoon garlic powder

1. Preheat the oven to 400°F (204°C). Line two large baking sheets with parchment paper. 2. Place the salmon on the first prepared baking sheet, making sure the fillets are evenly spaced. Spray the salmon with the cooking oil spray. Drizzle the lemon juice over each of the salmon fillets, then sprinkle the black pepper and garlic salt over each fillet. 3. Spread the broccoli out evenly on the second prepared baking sheet and spray the broccoli with cooking oil spray. Sprinkle the sea salt and garlic powder over the broccoli. 4. Place both baking sheets in the oven. Bake the salmon for 10 to 12 minutes, until it is light brown, depending on your preferred doneness and the thickness of the fillets. Bake the broccoli for 12 minutes, until the edges are slightly crispy. Serve the salmon and broccoli immediately.

Per Serving:
calorie: 353 | fat: 19g | protein: 37g | carbs: 9g | sugars: 2g | fiber: 3g | sodium: 406mg

Spicy Corn and Shrimp Salad in Avocado

Prep time: 10 minutes | Cook time: 0 minutes |

Serves 2

¼ cup mayonnaise
1 teaspoon sriracha (or to taste)
½ teaspoon lemon zest
¼ teaspoon sea salt
4 ounces cooked baby shrimp

½ cup cooked and cooled corn kernels
½ red bell pepper, seeded and chopped
1 avocado, halved lengthwise

1. In a medium bowl, combine the mayonnaise, sriracha, lemon zest, and salt. 2. Add the shrimp, corn, and bell pepper. Mix to combine. 3. Spoon the mixture into the avocado halves.

Per Serving:

calories: 354 | fat: 25g | protein: 17g | carbs: 21g | sugars: 2g | fiber: 9g | sodium: 600mg

Lemony Salmon

Prep time: 30 minutes | Cook time: 10 minutes |

Serves 4

1½ pounds (680 g) salmon steak
½ teaspoon grated lemon zest
Freshly cracked mixed peppercorns, to taste
⅓ cup lemon juice

Fresh chopped chives, for garnish
½ cup dry white wine
½ teaspoon fresh cilantro, chopped
Fine sea salt, to taste

1. To prepare the marinade, place all ingredients, except for salmon steak and chives, in a deep pan. Bring to a boil over medium-high flame until it has reduced by half. Allow it to cool down. 2. After that, allow salmon steak to marinate in the refrigerator approximately 40 minutes. Discard the marinade and transfer the fish steak to the preheated air fryer. 3. Air fry at 400ºF (204ºC) for 9 to 10 minutes. To finish, brush hot fish steaks with the reserved marinade, garnish with fresh chopped chives, and serve right away!

Per Serving:

calories: 244 | fat: 8g | protein: 35g | carbs: 3g | fiber: 0g | sodium: 128mg

Ahi Tuna Steaks

Prep time: 5 minutes | Cook time: 14 minutes |

Serves 2

2 (6 ounces / 170 g) ahi tuna steaks
2 tablespoons olive oil

3 tablespoons everything bagel seasoning

1. Drizzle both sides of each steak with olive oil. Place seasoning on a medium plate and press each side of tuna steaks into seasoning to form a thick layer. 2. Place steaks into ungreased air fryer basket. Adjust the temperature to 400ºF (204ºC) and air fry for 14 minutes, turning steaks halfway through cooking. Steaks will be done when internal temperature is at least 145ºF (63ºC) for well-done. Serve warm.

Per Serving:

calories: 305 | fat: 14g | protein: 42g | carbs: 0g | fiber: 0g | sodium: 377mg

Ginger-Glazed Salmon and Broccoli

Prep time: 10 minutes | Cook time: 15 minutes |

Serves 4

Nonstick cooking spray
1 tablespoon low-sodium tamari or gluten-free soy sauce
Juice of 1 lemon
1 tablespoon honey
1 (1-inch) piece fresh ginger, grated
1 garlic clove, minced

1 pound salmon fillet
¼ teaspoon salt, divided
⅛ teaspoon freshly ground black pepper
2 broccoli heads, cut into florets
1 tablespoon extra-virgin olive oil

1. Preheat the oven to 400°F. Spray a baking sheet with nonstick cooking spray. 2. In a small bowl, mix the tamari, lemon juice, honey, ginger, and garlic. Set aside. 3. Place the salmon skin-side down on the prepared baking sheet. Season with ⅛ teaspoon of salt and the pepper. 4. In a large mixing bowl, toss the broccoli and olive oil. Season with the remaining ⅛ teaspoon of salt. Arrange in a single layer on the baking sheet next to the salmon. Bake for 15 to 20 minutes until the salmon flakes easily with a fork and the broccoli is fork-tender. 5. In a small pan over medium heat, bring the tamari-ginger mixture to a simmer and cook for 1 to 2 minutes until it just begins to thicken. 6. Drizzle the sauce over the salmon and serve.

Per Serving:

calories: 238 | fat: 11g | protein: 25g | carbs: 11g | sugars: 6g | fiber: 2g | sodium: 334mg

Salmon Fritters with Zucchini

Prep time: 15 minutes | Cook time: 12 minutes |

Serves 4

2 tablespoons almond flour
1 zucchini, grated
1 egg, beaten
6 ounces (170 g) salmon fillet,

diced
1 teaspoon avocado oil
½ teaspoon ground black pepper

1. Mix almond flour with zucchini, egg, salmon, and ground black pepper. 2. Then make the fritters from the salmon mixture. 3. Sprinkle the air fryer basket with avocado oil and put the fritters inside. 4. Cook the fritters at 375ºF (191ºC) for 6 minutes per side.

Per Serving:

calories: 102 | fat: 4g | protein: 11g | carbs: 4g | fiber: 1g | sodium: 52mg

Crab-Stuffed Avocado Boats

Prep time: 5 minutes | Cook time: 7 minutes | Serves 4

2 medium avocados, halved and pitted
8 ounces (227 g) cooked crab meat

¼ teaspoon Old Bay seasoning
2 tablespoons peeled and diced yellow onion
2 tablespoons mayonnaise

1. Scoop out avocado flesh in each avocado half, leaving ½ inch around edges to form a shell. Chop scooped-out avocado. 2. In a medium bowl, combine crab meat, Old Bay seasoning, onion, mayonnaise, and chopped avocado. Place ¼ mixture into each avocado shell. 3. Place avocado boats into ungreased air fryer basket. Adjust the temperature to 350ºF (177ºC) and air fry for 7 minutes. Avocado will be browned on the top and mixture will be bubbling when done. Serve warm.

Per Serving:

calories: 226 | fat: 17g | protein: 12g | carbs: 10g | sugars: 1g | fiber: 7g | sodium: 239mg

Sea Bass with Ginger Sauce

Prep time: 5 minutes | Cook time: 15 minutes | Serves 2

Two 4 ounces sea bass filets
1 tablespoon extra-virgin olive oil
2 tablespoons minced fresh ginger

2 garlic cloves, minced
⅓ cup minced scallions
4 teaspoons chopped cilantro
1 tablespoon light soy sauce

1. In a medium steamer, add water and bring to a boil. Arrange the filets on the steamer rack. Cover, and steam for 6–8 minutes. 2. Meanwhile, in a small skillet, heat the oil over medium-high heat. Add the ginger and garlic, and sauté for 2 to 3 minutes. 3. Transfer the steamed filets to a platter. Pour the ginger oil over the filets, and top with scallions, cilantro, and soy sauce.

Per Serving:

calories: 207 | fat: 11g | protein: 22g | carbs: 5g | sugars: 2g | fiber: 1g | sodium: 202mg

Lemon Pepper Salmon

Prep time: 5 minutes | Cook time: 20 minutes | Serves 4

Avocado oil cooking spray
20 Brussels sprouts, halved lengthwise
4 (4 ounces) skinless salmon fillets
½ teaspoon garlic powder

½ teaspoon freshly ground black pepper
¼ teaspoon salt
2 teaspoons freshly squeezed lemon juice

1. Heat a large skillet over medium-low heat. When hot, coat the cooking surface with cooking spray, and put the Brussels sprouts cut-side down in the skillet. Cover and cook for 5 minutes. 2. Meanwhile, season both sides of the salmon with the garlic powder, pepper, and salt. 3. Flip the Brussels sprouts, and move them to one side of the skillet. Add the salmon and cook, uncovered, for 4 to 6 minutes. 4. Check the Brussels sprouts. When they are tender, remove them from the skillet and set them aside. 5. Flip the salmon fillets. Cook for 4 to 6 more minutes, or until the salmon is opaque and flakes easily with a fork. Remove the salmon from the skillet, and let it rest for 5 minutes. 6. Divide the Brussels sprouts into four equal portions and add 1 salmon fillet to each portion. Sprinkle the lemon juice on top and serve.

Per Serving:

calories: 163 | fat: 7g | protein: 23g | carbs: 1g | sugars: 0g | fiber: 0g | sodium: 167mg

Baked Garlic Scampi

Prep time: 5 minutes | Cook time: 10 minutes | Serves 4

1 tablespoon extra-virgin olive oil
¼ teaspoon salt
7 garlic cloves, crushed
2 tablespoons chopped fresh

parsley, divided
1 pound large shrimp, shelled (with tails left on) and deveined
Juice and zest of 1 lemon
2 cups baby arugula

1. Preheat the oven to 350 degrees. Grease a 13-x-9-x-2-inch baking pan with the olive oil. Add the salt, garlic, and 1 tablespoon of the parsley in a medium bowl; mix well, and set aside. 2. Arrange the shrimp in a single layer in the baking pan, and bake for 3 minutes, uncovered. Turn the shrimp, and sprinkle with the lemon peel, lemon juice, and the remaining 1 tablespoon of parsley. Continue to bake 1–2 minutes more until the shrimp are bright pink and tender. 3. Remove the shrimp from the oven. Place the arugula on a serving platter, and top with the shrimp. Spoon the garlic mixture over the shrimp and arugula, and serve.

Per Serving:

calories: 140 | fat: 4g | protein: 23g | carbs: 3g | sugars: 1g | fiber: 0g | sodium: 285mg

Lime Lobster Tails

Prep time: 10 minutes | Cook time: 6 minutes | Serves 4

4 lobster tails, peeled
2 tablespoons lime juice

½ teaspoon dried basil
½ teaspoon coconut oil, melted

1. Mix lobster tails with lime juice, dried basil, and coconut oil. 2. Put the lobster tails in the air fryer and cook at 380ºF (193ºC) for 6 minutes.

Per Serving:

calories: 123 | fat: 2g | protein: 25g | carbs: 1g | fiber: 0g | sodium: 635mg

Tuna Steak

Prep time: 10 minutes | Cook time: 12 minutes |

Serves 4

1 pound (454 g) tuna steaks, boneless and cubed
1 tablespoon mustard

1 tablespoon avocado oil
1 tablespoon apple cider vinegar

1. Mix avocado oil with mustard and apple cider vinegar. 2. Then brush tuna steaks with mustard mixture and put in the air fryer basket. 3. Cook the fish at 360ºF (182ºC) for 6 minutes per side.

Per Serving:

calories: 197 | fat: 9g | protein: 27g | carbs: 0g | fiber: 0g | sodium: 87mg

Roasted Salmon with Honey-Mustard Sauce

Prep time: 5 minutes | Cook time: 20 minutes |

Serves 4

Nonstick cooking spray
2 tablespoons whole-grain mustard
1 tablespoon honey
2 garlic cloves, minced

¼ teaspoon salt
¼ teaspoon freshly ground black pepper
1 pound salmon fillet

1. Preheat the oven to 425°F. Spray a baking sheet with nonstick cooking spray. 2. In a small bowl, whisk together the mustard, honey, garlic, salt, and pepper. 3. Place the salmon fillet on the prepared baking sheet, skin-side down. Spoon the sauce onto the salmon and spread evenly. 4. Roast for 15 to 20 minutes, depending on the thickness of the fillet, until the flesh flakes easily.

Per Serving:

calories: 186 | fat: 7g | protein: 23g | carbs: 6g | sugars: 4g | fiber: 0g | sodium: 312mg

Almond Catfish

Prep time: 10 minutes | Cook time: 12 minutes |

Serves 4

2 pounds (907 g) catfish fillet
½ cup almond flour
2 eggs, beaten

1 teaspoon salt
1 teaspoon avocado oil

1. Sprinkle the catfish fillet with salt and dip in the eggs. 2. Then coat the fish in the almond flour and put in the air fryer basket. Sprinkle the fish with avocado oil. 3. Cook the fish for 6 minutes per side at 380ºF (193ºC).

Per Serving:

calories: 308 | fat: 10g | protein: 42g | carbs: 11g | sugars: 0g | fiber: 2g | sodium: 610mg

Savory Shrimp

Prep time: 5 minutes | Cook time: 8 to 10 minutes |

Serves 4

1 pound (454 g) fresh large shrimp, peeled and deveined
1 tablespoon avocado oil
2 teaspoons minced garlic, divided
½ teaspoon red pepper flakes

Sea salt and freshly ground black pepper, to taste
2 tablespoons unsalted butter, melted
2 tablespoons chopped fresh parsley

1. Place the shrimp in a large bowl and toss with the avocado oil, 1 teaspoon of minced garlic, and red pepper flakes. Season with salt and pepper. 2. Set the air fryer to 350ºF (177ºC). Arrange the shrimp in a single layer in the air fryer basket, working in batches if necessary. Cook for 6 minutes. Flip the shrimp and cook for 2 to 4 minutes more, until the internal temperature of the shrimp reaches 120ºF (49ºC). (The time it takes to cook will depend on the size of the shrimp.) 3. While the shrimp are cooking, melt the butter in a small saucepan over medium heat and stir in the remaining 1 teaspoon of garlic. 4. Transfer the cooked shrimp to a large bowl, add the garlic butter, and toss well. Top with the parsley and serve warm.

Per Serving:

calories: 182 | fat: 10g | protein: 23g | carbs: 1g | sugars: 0g | fiber: 0g | sodium: 127mg

Greek Scampi

Prep time: 10 minutes | Cook time: 5 minutes |

Serves 2

2 garlic cloves, minced
2 tablespoons extra-virgin olive oil
½ pound shrimp, peeled, deveined, and thoroughly rinsed
1 cup diced tomatoes
½ cup nonfat ricotta cheese
6 Kalamata olives

Juice of ½ lemon
2 teaspoons chopped fresh dill, or ¾ teaspoon dried
Dash salt
Dash freshly ground black pepper
Lemon wedges, for garnish

1. In a large skillet set over medium heat, sauté the garlic in the olive oil for 30 seconds. 2. Add the shrimp. Cook for 1 minute. 3. Add the tomatoes, ricotta cheese, olives, lemon juice, and dill. Reduce the heat to low. Simmer for 5 to 10 minutes, stirring so the shrimp cook on both sides. When the shrimp are pink and the tomatoes and ricotta have made a sauce, the dish is ready. 4. Sprinkle with salt and pepper. 5. Serve immediately, garnished with lemon wedges.

Per Serving:

calories: 345 | fat: 21g | protein: 31g | carbs: 11g | sugars: 3g | fiber: 2g | sodium: 406mg

Ginger-Garlic Cod Cooked in Paper

Prep time: 10 minutes | Cook time: 15 minutes |

Serves 4

1 chard bunch, stemmed, leaves and stems cut into thin strips
1 red bell pepper, seeded and cut into strips
1 pound cod fillets cut into 4 pieces
1 tablespoon grated fresh ginger
3 garlic cloves, minced
2 tablespoons white wine vinegar
2 tablespoons low-sodium tamari or gluten-free soy sauce
1 tablespoon honey

1. Preheat the oven to 425°F. 2. Cut four pieces of parchment paper, each about 16 inches wide. Lay the four pieces out on a large workspace. 3. On each piece of paper, arrange a small pile of chard leaves and stems, topped by several strips of bell pepper. Top with a piece of cod. 4. In a small bowl, mix the ginger, garlic, vinegar, tamari, and honey. Top each piece of fish with one-fourth of the mixture. 5. Fold the parchment paper over so the edges overlap. Fold the edges over several times to secure the fish in the packets. Carefully place the packets on a large baking sheet. 6. Bake for 12 minutes. Carefully open the packets, allowing steam to escape, and serve.

Per Serving:

calories: 118 | fat: 1g | protein: 19g | carbs: 9g | sugars: 6g | fiber: 1g | sodium: 715mg

Baked Salmon with Lemon Sauce

Prep time: 10 minutes | Cook time: 15 minutes |

Serves 4

4 (5 ounces) salmon fillets
Sea salt
Freshly ground black pepper
1 tablespoon extra-virgin olive oil
½ cup low-sodium vegetable broth
Juice and zest of 1 lemon
1 teaspoon chopped fresh thyme
½ cup fat-free sour cream
1 teaspoon honey
1 tablespoon chopped fresh chives

1. Preheat the oven to 400°F. 2. Season the salmon lightly on both sides with salt and pepper. 3. Place a large ovenproof skillet over medium-high heat and add the olive oil. 4. Sear the salmon fillets on both sides until golden, about 3 minutes per side. 5. Transfer the salmon to a baking dish and bake until it is just cooked through, about 10 minutes. 6. While the salmon is baking, whisk together the vegetable broth, lemon juice, zest, and thyme in a small saucepan over medium-high heat until the liquid reduces by about one-quarter, about 5 minutes. 7. Whisk in the sour cream and honey. 8. Stir in the chives and serve the sauce over the salmon.

Per Serving:

calories: 243 | fat: 10g | protein: 30g | carbs: 8g | sugars: 2g | fiber: 1g | sodium: 216mg

Catfish with Corn and Pepper Relish

Prep time: 10 minutes | Cook time: 10 minutes |

Serves 4

3 tablespoons extra-virgin olive oil, divided
4 (5 ounces) catfish fillets
¼ teaspoon salt
¼ teaspoon freshly ground black pepper
1 (15 ounces) can low-sodium
black beans, drained and rinsed
1 cup frozen corn
1 medium red bell pepper, diced
1 tablespoon apple cider vinegar
3 tablespoons chopped scallions

1. Use 1½ tablespoons of oil to coat both sides of the catfish fillets, then season the fillets with the salt and pepper. 2. Heat a small saucepan over medium-high heat. Put the remaining 1½ tablespoons of oil, beans, corn, bell pepper, and vinegar in the pan and stir. Cover and cook for 5 minutes. 3. Place the catfish fillets on top of the relish mixture and cover. Cook for 5 to 7 minutes. 4. Serve each catfish fillet with one-quarter of the relish and top with the scallions.

Per Serving:

calories: 379 | fat: 15g | protein: 32g | carbs: 31g | sugars: 2g | fiber: 10g | sodium: 366mg

Five-Spice Tilapia

Prep time: 15 minutes | Cook time: 5 minutes |

Serves 2

8 ounces tilapia fillets
½ teaspoon Chinese five-spice powder
2 tablespoons reduced-sodium soy sauce
1 tablespoon granulated stevia
2 teaspoons extra-virgin olive oil
2 cups sugar snap peas
2 scallions, thinly sliced

1. Sprinkle both sides of the fillets with the Chinese five-spice powder. 2. In a small bowl, stir together the soy sauce and stevia. Set aside. 3. In a large nonstick skillet set over medium-high heat, heat the olive oil. 4. Add the tilapia. Cook for about 2 minutes, or until the outer edges are opaque. Reduce the heat to medium. Turn the fish over. Stir the soy mixture and pour into the skillet. 5. Add the sugar snap peas. Bring the sauce to a boil. Cook for about 2 minutes, or until the fish is cooked through, the sauce thickens, and the peas are bright green. 6. Add scallions. Remove from the heat. 7. Serve the fish and the sugar snap peas drizzled with the pan sauce.

Per Serving:

calories: 260 | fat: 10g | protein: 27g | carbs: 18g | sugars: 13g | fiber: 3g | sodium: 304mg

Scallops in Lemon-Butter Sauce

Prep time: 10 minutes | Cook time: 6 minutes |

Serves 2

8 large dry sea scallops (about ¾ pound / 340 g)
Salt and freshly ground black pepper, to taste
2 tablespoons olive oil
2 tablespoons unsalted butter, melted

2 tablespoons chopped flat-leaf parsley
1 tablespoon fresh lemon juice
2 teaspoons capers, drained and chopped
1 teaspoon grated lemon zest
1 clove garlic, minced

1. Preheat the air fryer to 400°F (204°C). 2. Use a paper towel to pat the scallops dry. Sprinkle lightly with salt and pepper. Brush with the olive oil. Arrange the scallops in a single layer in the air fryer basket. Pausing halfway through the cooking time to turn the scallops, air fry for about 6 minutes until firm and opaque. 3. Meanwhile, in a small bowl, combine the oil, butter, parsley, lemon juice, capers, lemon zest, and garlic. Drizzle over the scallops just before serving.

Per Serving:

calories: 304 | fat: 22g | protein: 21g | carbs: 5g | net carbs: 4g | fiber: 1g

Rainbow Salmon Kebabs

Prep time: 10 minutes | Cook time: 8 minutes |

Serves 2

6 ounces (170 g) boneless, skinless salmon, cut into 1-inch cubes
¼ medium red onion, peeled and cut into 1-inch pieces
½ medium yellow bell pepper, seeded and cut into 1-inch

pieces
½ medium zucchini, trimmed and cut into ½-inch slices
1 tablespoon olive oil
½ teaspoon salt
¼ teaspoon ground black pepper

1. Using one (6-inch) skewer, skewer 1 piece salmon, then 1 piece onion, 1 piece bell pepper, and finally 1 piece zucchini. Repeat this pattern with additional skewers to make four kebabs total. Drizzle with olive oil and sprinkle with salt and black pepper. 2. Place kebabs into ungreased air fryer basket. Adjust the temperature to 400°F (204°C) and air fry for 8 minutes, turning kebabs halfway through cooking. Salmon will easily flake and have an internal temperature of at least 145°F (63°C) when done; vegetables will be tender. Serve warm.

Per Serving:

calories: 195 | fat: 11g | protein: 19g | carbs: 6g | fiber: 2g | sodium: 651mg

Spicy Citrus Sole

Prep time: 10 minutes | Cook time: 10 minutes |

Serves 4

1 teaspoon chili powder
1 teaspoon garlic powder
½ teaspoon lime zest
½ teaspoon lemon zest
¼ teaspoon freshly ground black pepper
¼ teaspoon smoked paprika

Pinch sea salt
4 (6 ounces) sole fillets, patted dry
1 tablespoon extra-virgin olive oil
2 teaspoons freshly squeezed lime juice

1. Preheat the oven to 450°F. 2. Line a baking sheet with aluminum foil and set it aside. 3. In a small bowl, stir together the chili powder, garlic powder, lime zest, lemon zest, pepper, paprika, and salt until well mixed. 4. Pat the fish fillets dry with paper towels, place them on the baking sheet, and rub them lightly all over with the spice mixture. 5. Drizzle the olive oil and lime juice on the top of the fish. 6. Bake until the fish flakes when pressed lightly with a fork, about 8 minutes. Serve immediately.

Per Serving:

calories: 155 | fat: 7g | protein: 21g | carbs: 1g | sugars: 0g | fiber: 1g | sodium: 524mg

Herb-Crusted Halibut

Prep time: 10 minutes | Cook time: 20 minutes |

Serves 4

4 (5 ounces) halibut fillets
Extra-virgin olive oil, for brushing
½ cup coarsely ground unsalted pistachios
1 tablespoon chopped fresh

parsley
1 teaspoon chopped fresh thyme
1 teaspoon chopped fresh basil
Pinch sea salt
Pinch freshly ground black pepper

1. Preheat the oven to 350°F. 2. Line a baking sheet with parchment paper. 3. Pat the halibut fillets dry with a paper towel and place them on the baking sheet. 4. Brush the halibut generously with olive oil. 5. In a small bowl, stir together the pistachios, parsley, thyme, basil, salt, and pepper. 6. Spoon the nut and herb mixture evenly on the fish, spreading it out so the tops of the fillets are covered. 7. Bake the halibut until it flakes when pressed with a fork, about 20 minutes. 8. Serve immediately.

Per Serving:

calories: 351 | fat: 27g | protein: 24g | carbs: 4g | sugars: 1g | fiber: 2g | sodium: 214mg

Baked Monkfish

Prep time: 20 minutes | Cook time: 12 minutes | Serves 2

2 teaspoons olive oil
1 cup celery, sliced
2 bell peppers, sliced
1 teaspoon dried thyme
½ teaspoon dried marjoram
½ teaspoon dried rosemary

2 monkfish fillets
1 tablespoon coconut aminos
2 tablespoons lime juice
Coarse salt and ground black pepper, to taste
1 teaspoon cayenne pepper
½ cup Kalamata olives, pitted and sliced

1. In a nonstick skillet, heat the olive oil for 1 minute. Once hot, sauté the celery and peppers until tender, about 4 minutes. Sprinkle with thyme, marjoram, and rosemary and set aside. 2. Toss the fish fillets with the coconut aminos, lime juice, salt, black pepper, and cayenne pepper. Place the fish fillets in the lightly greased air fryer basket and bake at 390°F (199°C) for 8 minutes. 3. Turn them over, add the olives, and cook an additional 4 minutes. Serve with the sautéed vegetables on the side. Bon appétit!

Per Serving:

calories: 263 | fat: 11g | protein: 27g | carbs: 13g | fiber: 5g | sodium: 332mg

Cod with Jalapeño

Prep time: 5 minutes | Cook time: 14 minutes | Serves 4

4 cod fillets, boneless
1 jalapeño, minced

1 tablespoon avocado oil
½ teaspoon minced garlic

1. In the shallow bowl, mix minced jalapeño, avocado oil, and minced garlic. 2. Put the cod fillets in the air fryer basket in one layer and top with minced jalapeño mixture. 3. Cook the fish at 365°F (185°C) for 7 minutes per side.

Per Serving:

calories: 222 | fat: 5g | protein: 41g | carbs: 0g | fiber: 0g | sodium: 125mg

Chapter 7 Snacks and Appetizers

Ground Turkey Lettuce Cups

Prep time: 5 minutes | Cook time: 30 minutes |
Serves 8

3 tablespoons water
2 tablespoons soy sauce, tamari, or coconut aminos
3 tablespoons fresh lime juice
2 teaspoons Sriracha, plus more for serving
2 tablespoons cold-pressed avocado oil
2 teaspoons toasted sesame oil
4 garlic cloves, minced
1-inch piece fresh ginger, peeled and minced
2 carrots, diced
2 celery stalks, diced

1 yellow onion, diced
2 pounds 93 percent lean ground turkey
½ teaspoon fine sea salt
Two 8-ounce cans sliced water chestnuts, drained and chopped
1 tablespoon cornstarch
2 hearts romaine lettuce or 2 heads butter lettuce, leaves separated
½ cup roasted cashews (whole or halves and pieces), chopped
1 cup loosely packed fresh cilantro leaves

1. In a small bowl, combine the water, soy sauce, 2 tablespoons of the lime juice, and the Sriracha and mix well. Set aside. 2. Select the Sauté setting on the Instant Pot and heat the avocado oil, sesame oil, garlic, and ginger for 2 minutes, until the garlic is bubbling but not browned. Add the carrots, celery, and onion and sauté for about 3 minutes, until the onion begins to soften. 3. Add the turkey and salt and sauté, using a wooden spoon or spatula to break up the meat as it cooks, for about 5 minutes, until cooked through and no streaks of pink remain. Add the water chestnuts and soy sauce mixture and stir to combine, working quickly so not too much steam escapes. 4. Secure the lid and set the Pressure Release to Sealing. Press the Cancel button to reset the cooking program, then select the Pressure Cook or Manual setting and set the cooking time for 5 minutes at high pressure. (The pot will take about 10 minutes to come up to pressure before the cooking program begins.) 5. When the cooking program ends, perform a quick pressure release by moving the Pressure Release to Venting, or let the pressure release naturally. Open the pot. 6. In a small bowl, stir together the remaining 1 tablespoon lime juice and the cornstarch, add the mixture to the pot, and stir to combine. Press the Cancel button to reset the cooking program, then select the Sauté setting. Let the mixture come to a boil and thicken, stirring often, for about 2 minutes, then press the Cancel button to turn off the pot. 7. Spoon the turkey mixture onto the lettuce leaves and sprinkle the cashews and cilantro on top. Serve right away, with additional Sriracha at the table.

Per Serving:
calories: 127 | fat: 7g | protein: 6g | carbs: 10g | sugars: 2g | fiber: 3g | sodium: 392mg

Southern Boiled Peanuts

Prep time: 5 minutes | Cook time: 1 hour 20 minutes
| Makes 8 cups

1 pound raw jumbo peanuts in the shell
3 tablespoons fine sea salt

1. Remove the inner pot from the Instant Pot and add the peanuts to it. Cover the peanuts with water and use your hands to agitate them, loosening any dirt. Drain the peanuts in a colander, rinse out the pot, and return the peanuts to it. Return the inner pot to the Instant Pot housing. 2. Add the salt and 9 cups water to the pot and stir to dissolve the salt. Select a salad plate just small enough to fit inside the pot and set it on top of the peanuts to weight them down, submerging them all in the water. 3. Secure the lid and set the Pressure Release to Sealing. Select the Steam setting and set the cooking time for 1 hour at low pressure. (The pot will take about 20 minutes to come up to pressure before the cooking program begins.) 4. When the cooking program ends, let the pressure release naturally (this will take about 1 hour). Open the pot and, wearing heat-resistant mitts, remove the inner pot from the housing. Let the peanuts cool to room temperature in the brine (this will take about 1½ hours). 5. Serve at room temperature or chilled. Transfer the peanuts with their brine to an airtight container and refrigerate for up to 1 week.

Per Serving:
calories: 306 | fat: 17g | protein: 26g | carbs: 12g | sugars: 2g | fiber: 4g | sodium: 303mg

Guacamole with Jicama

Prep time: 5 minutes | Cook time: 0 minutes | Serves 4

1 avocado, cut into cubes
Juice of ½ lime
2 tablespoons finely chopped red onion
2 tablespoons chopped fresh

cilantro
1 garlic clove, minced
¼ teaspoon sea salt
1 cup sliced jicama

1. In a small bowl, combine the avocado, lime juice, onion, cilantro, garlic, and salt. Mash lightly with a fork. 2. Serve with the jicama for dipping.

Per Serving:
calorie: 97 | fat: 7g | protein: 1g | carbs: 8g | sugars: 1g | fiber: 5g | sodium: 151mg

Creamy Jalapeño Chicken Dip

Prep time: 5 minutes | Cook time: 12 minutes |
Serves 10

1 pound boneless chicken breast
8 ounces low-fat cream cheese
3 jalapeños, seeded and sliced
½ cup water

8 ounces reduced-fat shredded
cheddar cheese
¾ cup low-fat sour cream

1. Place the chicken, cream cheese, jalapeños, and water in the inner pot of the Instant Pot. 2. Secure the lid so it's locked and turn the vent to sealing. 3. Press Manual and set the Instant Pot for 12 minutes on high pressure. 4. When cooking time is up, turn off Instant Pot, do a quick release of the remaining pressure, then remove lid. 5. Shred the chicken between 2 forks, either in the pot or on a cutting board, then place back in the inner pot. 6. Stir in the shredded cheese and sour cream.

Per Serving:

calories: 238 | fat: 13g | protein: 24g | carbs: 7g | sugars: 5g | fiber: 1g | sodium: 273mg

Roasted Carrot and Chickpea Dip

Prep time: 10 minutes | Cook time: 15 minutes |
Makes 4 cups

4 medium carrots, quartered
lengthwise
¼ cup plus 2 teaspoons extra-
virgin olive oil, divided
Pinch kosher salt
Pinch freshly ground black
pepper
1 (15 ounces) can chickpeas,
drained and rinsed
1 garlic clove, minced

1 red chile (optional)
Zest and juice of 1 lemon
2 tablespoons tahini
1 tablespoon harissa
½ teaspoon ground cumin
¼ teaspoon ground coriander
Pomegranate arils (seeds)
(optional)
Cilantro, chopped (optional)

1. Preheat the oven to 425°F. Line a baking sheet with parchment paper. 2. In a medium bowl, toss the carrots with 2 teaspoons of extra-virgin olive oil, the salt, and the pepper. Spread them in a single layer on the prepared baking sheet and roast until tender, about 15 minutes. Turn the carrots over halfway through. 3. Meanwhile, place the chickpeas, garlic, chile, lemon zest and juice, tahini, harissa, cumin, and coriander in a food processor. Set aside. Add the carrots to the processor when they are cooked. Pulse until the mixture is coarse. Scrape the bowl down, then turn the processor back on while you drizzle the remaining ¼ cup of extra-virgin olive oil through the feed tube of the machine. Adjust the seasonings as desired. If it's too thick, add water to thin. 4. Top with pomegranate seeds and chopped cilantro (if using,) and Serve with cut vegetables. 5. Store any leftovers in an airtight container in the refrigerator for up to 4 days.

Per Serving:

calorie: 141 | fat: 10g | protein: 3g | carbs: 12g | sugars: 3g | fiber: 3g | sodium: 93mg

Sweet Potato Oven Fries with Spicy Sour Cream

Prep time: 10 minutes | Cook time: 35 minutes |
Serves 4

1 teaspoon salt-free southwest
chipotle seasoning
2 large dark-orange sweet
potatoes (1 pound), peeled, cut
into ½-inch-thick slices

Olive oil cooking spray
½ cup reduced-fat sour cream
1 tablespoon sriracha sauce
1 tablespoon chopped fresh
cilantro

1 Heat oven to 425°F. Spray large cookie sheet with cooking spray. Place ¾ teaspoon of the seasoning in 1-gallon resealable food-storage plastic bag; add potatoes. Seal bag; shake until potatoes are evenly coated. Place potatoes in single layer on cookie sheet; spray lightly with cooking spray. Bake 20 minutes or until bottoms are golden brown. Turn potatoes; bake 10 to 15 minutes longer or until tender and bottoms are golden brown. 2 Meanwhile, in small bowl, stir sour cream, sriracha sauce, cilantro and remaining ¼ teaspoon seasoning; refrigerate until ready to serve. 3 Serve fries warm with spicy sour cream.

Per Serving:

calories: 120 | fat: 4g | protein: 2g | carbs: 20g | sugars: 7g | fiber: 3g | sodium: 140mg

Crab-Filled Mushrooms

Prep time: 5 minutes | Cook time: 25 minutes |
Serves 10

20 large fresh mushroom caps
6 ounces canned crabmeat,
rinsed, drained, and flaked
½ cup crushed whole-wheat
crackers
2 tablespoons chopped fresh
parsley
2 tablespoons finely chopped

green onion
⅛ teaspoon freshly ground
black pepper
¼ cup chopped pimiento
3 tablespoons extra-virgin olive
oil
10 tablespoons wheat germ

1. Preheat the oven to 350 degrees. Clean the mushrooms by dusting off any dirt on the cap with a mushroom brush or paper towel; remove the stems. 2. In a small mixing bowl, combine the crabmeat, crackers, parsley, onion, and pepper. 3. Place the mushroom caps in a 13-x-9-x-2-inch baking dish, crown side down. Stuff some of the crabmeat filling into each cap. Place a little pimiento on top of the filling. 4. Drizzle the olive oil over the caps and sprinkle each cap with ½ tablespoon wheat germ. Bake for 15 to 17 minutes. Transfer to a serving platter, and serve hot.

Per Serving:

calorie: 113 | fat: 6g | protein: 7g | carbs: 9g | sugars: 1g | fiber: 2g | sodium: 77mg

Ginger and Mint Dip with Fruit

Prep time: 20 minutes | Cook time: 0 minutes |

Serves 6

Dip
1¼ cups plain fat-free yogurt
¼ cup packed brown sugar
2 teaspoons chopped fresh mint leaves
2 teaspoons grated gingerroot

½ teaspoon grated lemon peel
Fruit Skewers
12 bamboo skewers (6 inch)
1 cup fresh raspberries
2 cups melon cubes (cantaloupe and/or honeydew)

1 In small bowl, mix dip ingredients with whisk until smooth. Cover; refrigerate at least 15 minutes to blend flavors. 2 On each skewer, alternately thread 3 raspberries and 2 melon cubes. Serve with dip.

Per Serving:

calories: 100 | fat: 0g | protein: 3g | carbs: 20g | sugars: 17g | fiber: 2g | sodium: 50mg

Kale Chip Nachos

Prep time: 10 minutes | Cook time: 20 minutes |

Serves 2 to 4

1 bunch kale, torn into bite-size pieces
3 tablespoons extra-virgin olive oil, divided
2 teaspoons ground cumin, divided
1 large sweet potato, cut into ¼-inch-thick rounds
1 (15 ounces) can black beans, rinsed and drained

½ teaspoon ground coriander
1 teaspoon chili powder
Optional Toppings
Avocado slices
Salsa
Jicama, sliced
Red onion, sliced
Fresh cilantro
Fresh chiles, minced
Fresh tomatoes, diced

1. Preheat the oven to 225°F. Line a baking sheet with parchment paper. 2. In a large bowl, toss the kale with 1 tablespoon of oil and 1 teaspoon of cumin. Use your hands to massage the kale and evenly distribute the oil. 3. Spread the kale in a single even layer on the prepared baking sheet. (You may need two lined baking sheets for this.) Bake for 15 minutes, then flip and toss, and bake for another 5 to 10 minutes. 4. Meanwhile, heat 1 tablespoon of oil in a large skillet over medium-high heat. Arrange the sweet potato rounds in a single layer in the skillet, cover, and let them cook until they begin to brown on the bottom, about 3 minutes. Flip the potatoes over and cook for 3 to 5 minutes more. 5. Add the black beans to the skillet with the remaining 1 tablespoon of oil, remaining 1 teaspoon of cumin, the coriander, and chili powder. Cook for 3 minutes, then set aside and keep warm if the kale is not yet finished baking. 6. Serve on a platter, starting with the kale as a base, topped with sweet potatoes, black beans, and finally, any optional toppings. 7. Store any leftovers in an airtight container in the refrigerator for 3 to 4 days.

Per Serving:

calorie: 296 | fat: 14g | protein: 10g | carbs: 34g | sugars: 2g | fiber: 12g | sodium: 599mg

Caprese Skewers

Prep time: 5 minutes | Cook time: 0 minutes | Serves 2

12 cherry tomatoes
12 basil leaves
8 (1-inch) pieces mozzarella

cheese
¼ cup Italian Vinaigrette (optional, for serving)

1. On each of 4 wooden skewers, thread the following: 1 tomato, 1 basil leaf, 1 piece of cheese, 1 tomato, 1 basil leaf, 1 piece of cheese, 1 basil leaf, 1 tomato. 2. Serve with the vinaigrette, if desired, for dipping.

Per Serving:

calorie: 475 | fat: 21g | protein: 39g | carbs: 38g | sugars: 24g | fiber: 11g | sodium: 63mg

Garlic Kale Chips

Prep time: 5 minutes | Cook time: 15 minutes |

Serves 1

1 (8-ounce) bunch kale, trimmed and cut into 2-inch pieces
1 tablespoon extra-virgin olive oil

½ teaspoon sea salt
¼ teaspoon garlic powder
Pinch cayenne (optional, to taste)

1. Preheat the oven to 350°F. Line two baking sheets with parchment paper. 2. Wash the kale and pat it completely dry. 3. In a large bowl, toss the kale with the olive oil, sea salt, garlic powder, and cayenne, if using. 4. Spread the kale in a single layer on the prepared baking sheets. 5. Bake until crisp, 12 to 15 minutes, rotating the sheets once.

Per Serving:

calorie: 78 | fat: 5g | protein: 3g | carbs: 7g | sugars: 2g | fiber: 3g | sodium: 416mg

Cinnamon Toasted Pumpkin Seeds

Prep time: 5 minutes | Cook time: 45 minutes |

Serves 4

1 cup pumpkin seeds
2 tablespoons canola oil
1 teaspoon cinnamon

2 (1-gram) packets stevia
¼ teaspoon sea salt

1. Preheat the oven to 300°F. 2. In a bowl, toss the pumpkin seeds with the oil, cinnamon, stevia, and salt. 3. Spread the seeds in a single layer on a rimmed baking sheet. Bake until browned and fragrant, stirring once or twice, about 45 minutes.

Per Serving:

calorie: 233 | fat: 21g | protein: 9g | carbs: 5g | sugars: 0g | fiber: 2g | sodium: 151mg

Guacamole

Prep time: 5 minutes | Cook time: 5 minutes | Serves 8

2 large (8½ ounces) ripe
avocados, peeled, pits removed,
and mashed
½ cup chopped onion
2 medium jalapeño peppers,
seeded and chopped
2 tablespoons minced fresh
parsley
2 tablespoons fresh lime juice

⅛ teaspoon freshly ground
black pepper
2 medium tomatoes, finely
chopped
1 medium garlic clove, minced
1 tablespoon extra-virgin olive
oil
½ teaspoon salt

1. In a large mixing bowl, combine all ingredients, blending well.

Per Serving:
calorie: 107 | fat: 9g | protein: 1g | carbs: 7g | sugars: 2g | fiber: 4g |
sodium: 152mg

Fresh Dill Dip

Prep time: 5 minutes | Cook time: 5 minutes | Serves 6

1 cup plain fat-free yogurt
¼ teaspoon salt
¼ teaspoon freshly ground
black pepper
¼ cup minced parsley
2 tablespoons finely chopped

fresh chives
1 tablespoon finely chopped
fresh dill
1 tablespoon apple cider
vinegar

1. In a small bowl, combine all the ingredients. Chill for 2 to 4
hours. Serve with fresh cut vegetables.

Per Serving:
calorie: 20 | fat: 0g | protein: 2g | carbs: 3g | sugars: 2g | fiber: 0g |
sodium: 120mg

Lemon Artichokes

**Prep time: 5 minutes | Cook time: 5 to 15 minutes |
Serves 4**

4 artichokes
1 cup water

2 tablespoons lemon juice
1 teaspoon salt

1. Wash and trim artichokes by cutting off the stems flush with the
bottoms of the artichokes and by cutting ¾–1 inch off the tops.
Stand upright in the bottom of the inner pot of the Instant Pot. 2.
Pour water, lemon juice, and salt over artichokes. 3. Secure the lid
and make sure the vent is set to sealing. On Manual, set the Instant
Pot for 15 minutes for large artichokes, 10 minutes for medium
artichokes, or 5 minutes for small artichokes. 4. When cook time is
up, perform a quick release by releasing the pressure manually.

Per Serving:
calories: 60 | fat: 0g | protein: 4g | carbs: 13g | sugars: 1g | fiber: 6g |
sodium: 397mg

Cucumber Pâté

**Prep time: 10 minutes | Cook time: 20 minutes |
Serves 12**

1 large cucumber, peeled,
seeded, and quartered
1 small green bell pepper,
seeded and quartered
3 stalks celery, quartered
1 medium onion, quartered

1 cup low-fat cottage cheese
½ cup plain nonfat Greek
yogurt
1 package unflavored gelatin
¼ cup boiling water
¼ cup cold water

1. Spray a 5-cup mold or a 1½-quart mixing bowl with nonstick
cooking spray. 2. In a food processor, coarsely chop the cucumber,
green pepper, celery, and onion. Remove the vegetables from the
food processor and set aside. 3. In a food processor, combine the
cottage cheese and yogurt, and blend until smooth. 4. In a medium
bowl, dissolve the gelatin in the boiling water; slowly stir in the
cold water. Add the chopped vegetables and cottage cheese mixture,
and mix thoroughly. 5. Pour the mixture into the prepared mold
and refrigerate overnight or until firm. To serve, carefully invert the
mold onto a serving plate, and remove the mold. Surround the pâté
with assorted crackers, and serve.

Per Serving:
calorie: 57 | fat: 2g | protein: 6g | carbs: 3g | sugars: 2g | fiber: 1g |
sodium: 107mg

Vegetable Kabobs with Mustard Dip

**Prep time: 35 minutes | Cook time: 10 minutes |
Serves 9**

Dip
⅔ cup plain fat-free yogurt
⅓ cup fat-free sour cream
1 tablespoon finely chopped
fresh parsley
1 teaspoon onion powder
1 teaspoon garlic salt
1 tablespoon Dijon mustard
Kabobs

1 medium bell pepper, cut into
6 strips, then cut into thirds
1 medium zucchini, cut
diagonally into ½-inch slices
1 package (8 ounces) fresh
whole mushrooms
9 large cherry tomatoes
2 tablespoons olive or vegetable
oil

1 In small bowl, mix dip ingredients. Cover; refrigerate at least 1
hour. 2 Heat gas or charcoal grill. On 5 (12-inch) metal skewers,
thread vegetables so that one kind of vegetable is on the same
skewer (use 2 skewers for mushrooms); leave space between each
piece. Brush vegetables with oil. 3 Place skewers of bell pepper and
zucchini on grill over medium heat. Cover grill; cook 2 minutes.
Add skewers of mushrooms and tomatoes. Cover grill; cook 4 to
5 minutes, carefully turning every 2 minutes, until vegetables are
tender. Transfer vegetables from skewers to serving plate. Serve
with dip.

Per Serving:
calories: 60 | fat: 3.5g | protein: 2g | carbs: 6g | sugars: 3g | fiber: 1g
| sodium: 180mg

Turkey Rollups with Veggie Cream Cheese

Prep time: 10 minutes | Cook time: 0 minutes |

Serves 2

¼ cup cream cheese, at room temperature
2 tablespoons finely chopped red onion
2 tablespoons finely chopped red bell pepper

1 tablespoon chopped fresh chives
1 teaspoon Dijon mustard
1 garlic clove, minced
¼ teaspoon sea salt
6 slices deli turkey

1. In a small bowl, mix the cream cheese, red onion, bell pepper, chives, mustard, garlic, and salt. 2. Spread the mixture on the turkey slices and roll up.

Per Serving:

calorie: 146 | fat: 1g | protein: 24g | carbs: 8g | sugars: 6g | fiber: 1g | sodium: 572mg

Hummus with Chickpeas and Tahini Sauce

Prep time: 10 minutes | Cook time: 55 minutes |

Makes 4 cups

4 cups water
1 cup dried chickpeas
2½ teaspoons fine sea salt
½ cup tahini

3 tablespoons fresh lemon juice
1 garlic clove
¼ teaspoon ground cumin

1. Combine the water, chickpeas, and 1 teaspoon of the salt in the Instant Pot and stir to dissolve the salt. 2. Secure the lid and set the Pressure Release to Sealing. Select the Bean/Chili, Pressure Cook, or Manual setting and set the cooking time for 40 minutes at high pressure. (The pot will take about 15 minutes to come up to pressure before the cooking program begins.) 3. When the cooking program ends, let the pressure release naturally for 15 minutes, then move the Pressure Release to Venting to release any remaining steam. 4. Place a colander over a bowl. Open the pot and, wearing heat-resistant mitts, lift out the inner pot and drain the beans in the colander. Return the chickpeas to the inner pot and place it back in the Instant Pot housing on the Keep Warm setting. Reserve the cooking liquid. 5. In a blender or food processor, combine 1 cup of the cooking liquid, the tahini, lemon juice, garlic, cumin, and 1 teaspoon salt. Blend or process on high speed, stopping to scrape down the sides of the container as needed, for about 30 seconds, until smooth and a little fluffy. Scoop out and set aside ½ cup of this sauce for the topping. 6. Set aside ½ cup of the chickpeas for the topping. Add the remaining chickpeas to the tahini sauce in the blender or food processor along with ½ cup of the cooking liquid and the remaining ½ teaspoon salt. Blend or process on high speed, stopping to scrape down the sides of the container as needed, for about 1 minute, until very smooth. 7. Transfer the hummus to a shallow serving bowl. Spoon the reserved tahini mixture over the top, then sprinkle on the reserved chickpeas. The hummus will keep in an airtight container in the refrigerator for up to 3 days. Serve at room temperature or chilled.

Per Serving:

calories: 107 | fat: 5g | protein: 4g | carbs: 10g | sugars: 3g | fiber: 4g | sodium: 753mg

Zucchini Hummus Dip with Red Bell Peppers

Prep time: 10 minutes | Cook time: 0 minutes |

Serves 4

2 zucchini, chopped
3 garlic cloves
2 tablespoons extra-virgin olive oil
2 tablespoons tahini

Juice of 1 lemon
½ teaspoon sea salt
1 red bell pepper, seeded and cut into sticks

1. In a blender or food processor, combine the zucchini, garlic, olive oil, tahini, lemon juice, and salt. Blend until smooth. 2. Serve with the red bell pepper for dipping.

Per Serving:

calorie: 136 | fat: 11g | protein: 3g | carbs: 8g | sugars: 4g | fiber: 2g | sodium: 309mg

Candied Pecans

Prep time: 5 minutes | Cook time: 20 minutes |

Serves 10

4 cups raw pecans
1½ teaspoons liquid stevia
½ cup plus 1 tablespoon water, divided
1 teaspoon vanilla extract

1 teaspoon cinnamon
¼ teaspoon nutmeg
⅛ teaspoon ground ginger
⅛ teaspoon sea salt

1. Place the raw pecans, liquid stevia, 1 tablespoon water, vanilla, cinnamon, nutmeg, ground ginger, and sea salt into the inner pot of the Instant Pot. 2. Press the Sauté button on the Instant Pot and sauté the pecans and other ingredients until the pecans are soft. 3. Pour in the ½ cup water and secure the lid to the locked position. Set the vent to sealing. 4. Press Manual and set the Instant Pot for 15 minutes. 5. Preheat the oven to 350°F. 6. When cooking time is up, turn off the Instant Pot, then do a quick release. 7. Spread the pecans onto a greased, lined baking sheet. 8. Bake the pecans for 5 minutes or less in the oven, checking on them frequently so they do not burn.

Per Serving:

calories: 275 | fat: 28g | protein: 4g | carbs: 6g | sugars: 2g | fiber: 4g | sodium: 20mg

Cocoa Coated Almonds

Prep time: 5 minutes | Cook time: 15 minutes |

Serves 4

1 cup almonds
1 tablespoon cocoa powder

2 packets powdered stevia

1. Preheat the oven to 350°F. Line a baking sheet with parchment paper. 2. Spread the almonds in a single layer on the baking sheet. Bake for 5 minutes. 3. While the almonds bake, in a small bowl, mix the cocoa and stevia well. Add the hot almonds to the bowl. Toss to combine. 4. Return the almonds to the baking sheet and bake until fragrant, about 5 minutes more.

Per Serving:

calorie: 143 | fat: 12g | protein: 5g | carbs: 6g | sugars: 1g | fiber: 3g | sodium: 1mg

Peanut Butter Protein Bites

Prep time: 10 minutes | Cook time: 0 minutes |

Makes 16 Balls

½ cup sugar-free peanut butter
¼ cup (1 scoop) sugar-free peanut butter powder or sugar-free protein powder
2 tablespoons unsweetened

cocoa powder
2 tablespoons canned coconut milk (or more to adjust consistency)

1. In a bowl, mix all ingredients until well combined. 2. Roll into 16 balls. Refrigerate before serving.

Per Serving:

calorie: 59 | fat: 5g | protein: 3g | carbs: 2g | sugars: 1g | fiber: 1g | sodium: 4mg

Lemon Cream Fruit Dip

Prep time: 5 minutes | Cook time: 0 minutes | Serves 4

1 cup (200 g) plain nonfat Greek yogurt
¼ cup (28 g) coconut flour 1 tablespoon (15 ml) pure maple syrup

½ teaspoon pure vanilla extract
½ teaspoon pure almond extract
Zest of 1 medium lemon
Juice of ½ medium lemon

1. In a medium bowl, whisk together the yogurt, coconut flour, maple syrup, vanilla, almond extract, lemon zest, and lemon juice. Serve the dip with fruit or crackers.

Per Serving:

calorie: 80 | fat: 1g | protein: 7g | carbs: 10g | sugars: 6g | fiber: 3g | sodium: 37mg

No-Bake Coconut and Cashew Energy Bars

Prep time: 5 minutes | Cook time: 0 minutes | Makes

12 energy bars

1 cup (110 g) raw cashews
1 cup (80 g) unsweetened shredded coconut
½ cup (120 g) unsweetened nut

butter of choice
2 tablespoons (30 ml) pure maple syrup

1. Line an 8 x 8–inch (20 x 20–cm) baking pan with parchment paper. 2. In a large food processor, combine the cashews and coconut. Pulse them for 15 to 20 seconds to form a powder. 3. Add the nut butter and maple syrup and process until a doughy paste is formed, scraping down the sides if needed. 4. Spread the dough into the prepared baking pan. Cover the dough with another sheet of parchment paper and press it flat. 5. Freeze the dough for 1 hour. Cut the dough into bars.

Per Serving:

calorie: 169 | fat: 14g | protein: 4g | carbs: 10g | sugars: 3g | fiber: 2g | sodium: 6mg

Monterey Jack Cheese Quiche Squares

Prep time: 10 minutes | Cook time: 15 minutes |

Serves 12

4 egg whites
1 cup plus 2 tablespoons low-fat cottage cheese
¼ cup plus 2 tablespoons flour
¾ teaspoon baking powder
1 cup shredded reduced-fat Monterey Jack cheese

½ cup diced green chilies
1 red bell pepper, diced
1 cup lentils, cooked
1 tablespoon extra-virgin olive oil
Parsley sprigs

1. Preheat the oven to 350 degrees. 2. In a medium bowl, beat the egg whites and cottage cheese for 2 minutes, until smooth. 3. Add the flour and baking powder, and beat until smooth. Stir in the cheese, green chilies, red pepper, and lentils. 4. Coat a 9-inch-square pan with the olive oil, and pour in the egg mixture. Bake for 30–35 minutes, until firm. 5. Remove the quiche from the oven, and allow to cool for 10 minutes (it will be easier to cut). Cut into 12 squares and transfer to a platter, garnish with parsley sprigs, and serve.

Per Serving:

calorie: 104 | fat: 6g | protein: 8g | carbs: 4g | sugars: 0g | fiber: 0g | sodium: 215mg

Chicken Kabobs

Prep time: 5 minutes | Cook time: 20 minutes |

Serves 6

1 pound boneless, skinless chicken breast
3 tablespoons light soy sauce
One 1-inch cube of fresh ginger root, finely chopped
3 tablespoons extra-virgin olive

oil
3 tablespoons dry vermouth
1 large clove garlic, finely chopped
12 watercress sprigs
2 large lemons, cut into wedges

1. Cut the chicken into 1-inch cubes and place in a shallow bowl. 2. In a small bowl, combine the soy sauce, ginger root, oil, vermouth, and garlic and pour over the chicken. Cover the chicken, and let marinate for at least 1 hour (or overnight). 3. Thread the chicken onto 12 metal or wooden skewers (remember to soak wooden skewers in water before using). Grill or broil 6 inches from the heat source for 8 minutes, turning frequently. 4. Arrange the skewers on a platter and garnish with the watercress and lemon wedges. Serve hot with additional soy sauce, if desired.

Per Serving:

calorie: 187 | fat: 10g | protein: 18g | carbs: 4g | sugars: 2g | fiber: 1g | sodium: 158mg

Gruyere Apple Spread

Prep time: 5 minutes | Cook time: 5 minutes | Serves

20

4 ounces fat-free cream cheese, softened
½ cup low-fat cottage cheese
4 ounces Gruyere cheese
¼ teaspoon dry mustard
⅛ teaspoon freshly ground

black pepper
½ cup shredded apple (unpeeled)
2 tablespoons finely chopped pecans
2 teaspoons minced fresh chives

1. Place the cheeses in a food processor, and blend until smooth. Add the mustard and pepper, and blend for 30 seconds. 2. Transfer the mixture to a serving bowl, and fold in the apple and pecans. Sprinkle the dip with chives. 3. Cover, and refrigerate the mixture for 1–2 hours. Serve chilled with crackers, or stuff into celery stalks.

Per Serving:

calorie: 46 | fat: 3g | protein: 4g | carbs: 1g | sugars: 1g | fiber: 0g | sodium: 107mg

Spinach and Artichoke Dip

Prep time: 5 minutes | Cook time: 4 minutes | Serves

11

8 ounces low-fat cream cheese
10 ounces box frozen spinach
½ cup no-sodium chicken broth
14 ounces can artichoke hearts, drained
½ cup low-fat sour cream
½ cup low-fat mayo

3 cloves of garlic, minced
1 teaspoon onion powder
16 ounces reduced-fat shredded Parmesan cheese
8 ounces reduced-fat shredded mozzarella

1. Put all ingredients in the inner pot of the Instant Pot, except the Parmesan cheese and the mozzarella cheese. 2. Secure the lid and set vent to sealing. Place on Manual high pressure for 4 minutes. 3. Do a quick release of steam. 4. Immediately stir in the cheeses.

Per Serving:

calories: 288 | fat: 18g | protein: 19g | carbs: 15g | sugars: 3g | fiber: 3g | sodium: 1007mg

Creamy Spinach Dip

Prep time: 13 minutes | Cook time: 5 minutes |

Serves 11

8 ounces low-fat cream cheese
1 cup low-fat sour cream
½ cup finely chopped onion
½ cup no-sodium vegetable broth
5 cloves garlic, minced
½ teaspoon salt

¼ teaspoon black pepper
10 ounces frozen spinach
12 ounces reduced-fat shredded Monterey Jack cheese
12 ounces reduced-fat shredded Parmesan cheese

1. Add cream cheese, sour cream, onion, vegetable broth, garlic, salt, pepper, and spinach to the inner pot of the Instant Pot. 2. Secure lid, make sure vent is set to sealing, and set to the Bean/Chili setting on high pressure for 5 minutes. 3. When done, do a manual release. 4. Add the cheeses and mix well until creamy and well combined.

Per Serving:

calorie: 274 | fat: 18g | protein: 19g | carbs: 10g | sugars: 3g | fiber: 1g | sodium: 948mg

Chapter 8 Vegetables and Sides

Dijon Roast Cabbage

Prep time: 10 minutes | Cook time: 10 minutes |

Serves 4

1 small head cabbage, cored and sliced into 1-inch-thick slices
2 tablespoons olive oil, divided
½ teaspoon salt
1 tablespoon Dijon mustard
1 teaspoon apple cider vinegar
1 teaspoon granular erythritol

1. Drizzle each cabbage slice with 1 tablespoon olive oil, then sprinkle with salt. Place slices into ungreased air fryer basket, working in batches if needed. Adjust the temperature to 350°F (177°C) and air fry for 10 minutes. Cabbage will be tender and edges will begin to brown when done. 2. In a small bowl, whisk remaining olive oil with mustard, vinegar, and erythritol. Drizzle over cabbage in a large serving dish. Serve warm.

Per Serving:

calories: 110 | fat: 7g | protein: 3g | carbs: 11g | sugars: 5g | fiber: 3g | sodium: 392mg

Summer Squash Casserole

Prep time: 15 minutes | Cook time: 30 minutes |

Serves 8

1 tablespoon extra-virgin olive oil
6 yellow summer squash, thinly sliced
1 large portobello mushroom, thinly sliced
1 Vidalia onion, thinly sliced
1 cup shredded Parmesan
cheese, divided
1 cup shredded reduced-fat extra-sharp Cheddar cheese
½ cup whole-wheat bread crumbs
½ cup tri-color quinoa
1 tablespoon Creole seasoning

1. Preheat the oven to 350°F. 2. In a large cast iron pan, heat the oil over medium heat. 3. Add the squash, mushroom, and onion, and sauté for 7 to 10 minutes, or until softened. 4. Remove from the heat. Add ½ cup of Parmesan cheese and the Cheddar cheese and mix well. 5. In a small bowl, whisk the bread crumbs, quinoa, the remaining ½ cup of Parmesan, and the Creole seasoning together. Evenly distribute over the casserole. 6. Transfer the pan to the oven, and bake for 20 minutes, or until browned. Serve warm and enjoy.

Per Serving:

calories: 163 | fat: 7g | protein: 10g | carbs: 14g | sugars: 1g | fiber: 2g | sodium: 484mg

Spaghetti Squash with Sun-Dried Tomatoes

Prep time: 20 minutes | Cook time: 1hour | Serves 4

1 spaghetti squash, halved and seeded
3 teaspoons extra-virgin olive oil, divided
¼ sweet onion, chopped
1 teaspoon minced garlic
2 cups fresh spinach
¼ cup chopped sun-dried tomatoes
¼ cup roasted, shelled sunflower seeds
Juice of ½ lemon
Sea salt
Freshly ground black pepper

1. Preheat the oven to 350°F. Line a baking sheet with parchment paper. 2. Place the squash on the baking sheet and brush the cut edges with 2 teaspoons of olive oil. 3. Bake the squash until it is tender and separates into strands with a fork, about 1 hour. 4. Let the squash cool for 5 minutes then use a fork to scrape out the strands from both halves of the squash. Cover the squash strands and set them aside. 5. Place a large skillet over medium-high heat and add the remaining 1 teaspoon of olive oil. Sauté the onion and garlic until softened and translucent, about 3 minutes. 6. Stir in the spinach and sun-dried tomatoes, and sauté until the spinach is wilted, about 4 minutes. 7. Remove the skillet from the heat and stir in the squash strands, sunflower seeds, and lemon juice. 8. Season with salt and pepper and serve warm.

Per Serving:

calories: 218 | fat: 10g | protein: 5g | carbs: 32g | sugars: 13g | fiber: 7g | sodium: 232mg

Best Brown Rice

Prep time: 5 minutes | Cook time: 22 minutes |

Serves 6 to 12

2 cups brown rice
2½ cups water

1. Rinse brown rice in a fine-mesh strainer. 2. Add rice and water to the inner pot of the Instant Pot. 3. Secure the lid and make sure vent is on sealing. 4. Use Manual setting and select 22 minutes cooking time on high pressure. 5. When cooking time is done, let the pressure release naturally for 10 minutes, then press Cancel and manually release any remaining pressure.

Per Serving:

calorie: 114 | fat: 1g | protein: 2g | carbs: 23g | sugars: 0g | fiber: 1g | sodium: 3mg

Simple Bibimbap

Prep time: 15 minutes | Cook time: 15 minutes |

Serves 2

4 teaspoons canola oil, divided
2½ cups cauliflower rice
2 cups fresh baby spinach
3 teaspoons low-sodium soy
sauce or tamari, divided
8 ounces mushrooms, thinly

sliced
2 large eggs
1 cup bean sprouts, rinsed
1 cup kimchi
½ cup shredded carrots

1. Heat 1 teaspoon of canola oil in a medium skillet and sauté the cauliflower rice, spinach, and 2 teaspoons of soy sauce until the greens are wilted, about 5 minutes. Put the vegetables in a small bowl and set aside. 2. Return the skillet to medium heat, add 2 teaspoons of vegetable oil and, when it's hot, add the mushrooms in a single layer and cook for 3 to 5 minutes, then stir and cook another 3 minutes or until mostly golden-brown in color. Put the mushrooms in a small bowl and toss them with the remaining 1 teaspoon of soy sauce. 3. Wipe out the skillet and heat the remaining 1 teaspoon of vegetable oil over low heat. Crack in the eggs and cook until the whites are set and the yolks begin to thicken but not harden, 4 to 5 minutes. 4. Assemble two bowls with cauliflower rice and spinach at the bottom. Then arrange each ingredient separately around the rim of the bowl: bean sprouts, mushrooms, kimchi, and shredded carrots, with the egg placed in the center, and serve.

Per Serving:

calories: 275 | fat: 16g | protein: 20g | carbs: 20g | sugars: 8g | fiber: 8g | sodium: 518mg

Mushroom Cassoulets

Prep time: 5 minutes | Cook time: 30 minutes |

Serves 6

1 pound mushrooms, sliced
½ cup lentils, cooked
1 medium onion, chopped
1 cup low-sodium chicken
broth
1 sprig thyme
1 bay leaf

Leaves from 1 celery stalk
2 tablespoons lemon juice
⅛ teaspoon freshly ground
black pepper
½ cup wheat germ
2 tablespoons extra-virgin olive
oil

1. Preheat the oven to 350 degrees. 2. In a saucepan, combine the mushrooms, lentils, onion, and chicken broth. Tie together the thyme, bay leaf, and celery leaves and add to the mushrooms. 3. Add the lemon juice and pepper, and bring to a boil. Boil until the liquid is reduced, about 10 minutes. Remove the bundle of herbs. 4. Divide the mushroom mixture equally into small ramekins. Mix the wheat germ and oil together, and sprinkle on top of each casserole. 5. Bake at 350 degrees for 20 minutes or until the tops are golden brown. Remove from the oven, and let cool slightly before serving. Add salt if desired.

Per Serving:

calories: 114 | fat: 6g | protein: 6g | carbs: 12g | sugars: 2g | fiber: 3g | sodium: 21mg

Smashed Cucumber Salad

Prep time: 10 minutes | Cook time: 0 minutes |

Serves 4 to 6

2 pounds mini cucumbers
(English or Persian), unpeeled
½ teaspoon kosher salt
1 tablespoon extra-virgin olive
oil

¾ teaspoon ground cumin
¼ teaspoon turmeric
Juice of 1 lime
½ cup cilantro leaves

1. Cut the cucumbers crosswise into 4-inch pieces and again in half lengthwise. 2. On a work surface, place one cucumber, flesh-side down. Place the side of the knife blade on the cucumber and carefully smash down lightly with your hand. Alternatively, put in a plastic bag, seal, and smash with a rolling pin or similar tool. Be careful not to break the bag. The skin of the cucumber should crack and flesh will break away. Repeat with all the cucumbers and cut the smashed pieces on a bias into bite-size pieces. 3. Transfer the cucumber pieces to a strainer and toss them with the salt. Allow the cucumbers to rest for at least 15 minutes. 4. Meanwhile, prepare the dressing by whisking together the extra-virgin olive oil, cumin, turmeric, and lime juice in a small bowl. 5. When the cucumbers are ready, shake them to remove any excess liquid. Transfer the cucumbers to a large bowl with the dressing and cilantro and toss to combine. Serve. 6. Store any leftovers in an airtight container in the refrigerator for up to 2 days.

Per Serving:

calories: 55 | fat: 3g | protein: 1g | carbs: 8g | sugars: 3g | fiber: 1g | sodium: 238mg

Zucchini on the Half Shell

Prep time: 15 minutes | Cook time: 30 minutes |

Serves 4 to 8

4 zucchini, cut lengthwise,
seeded, pulp removed
1 (13.4 ounces) box borlotti
beans, rinsed
½ onion, finely chopped
1 garlic clove, minced

1 cup coarsely chopped
tomatoes
2 teaspoons Creole seasoning
½ cup grated reduced-fat
Cheddar cheese

1. Preheat the oven to 350°F. 2. Arrange the zucchini on a rimmed baking sheet in a single layer, cavity-side up. 3. Transfer the baking sheet to the oven, and bake for 10 minutes, or until the exterior of the zucchini is soft. 4. Meanwhile, in a small pan, combine the beans, onion, garlic, tomatoes, and Creole seasoning. Cook over medium heat, stirring often, for 3 to 5 minutes, or until the onion and garlic are translucent. Remove from the heat. 5. Remove the zucchini from the oven, and spoon the tomato and bean mixture into the cavities. 6. Sprinkle 1 tablespoon of cheese on top of each stuffed zucchini. 7. Return the baking sheet to the oven and cook for 10 to 15 minutes, or until the cheese is melted and golden brown. Serve warm and enjoy.

Per Serving:

calories: 63 | fat: 1g | protein: 5g | carbs: 9g | sugars: 5g | fiber: 3g | sodium: 177mg

Classic Oven-Roasted Carrots

Prep time: 10 minutes | Cook time: 15 minutes |

Serves 4

1½ pounds (680 g) large
carrots, trimmed and washed
Avocado oil spray, as needed

¼ teaspoon sea salt
1 tablespoon (3 g) dried
rosemary

1. Preheat the oven to 400°F (204°C). Line a large baking sheet with parchment paper. 2. Arrange the carrots on the prepared baking sheet, making sure there is at least ½ inch (13 mm) between each of them. 3. Generously spray the carrots with the avocado oil spray, and then sprinkle them with the sea salt and rosemary. Roast the carrots for 15 minutes, or until they are fork-tender.

Per Serving:

calorie: 72 | fat: 1g | protein: 2g | carbs: 17g | sugars: 8g | fiber: 5g | sodium: 263mg

Cauliflower "Mashed Potatoes"

Prep time: 5 minutes | Cook time: 0 minutes | Serves 2

2 cups cooked cauliflower
florets
1 tablespoon plain nonfat Greek
yogurt
½ teaspoon extra-virgin olive

oil
Salt, to season
Freshly ground black pepper, to
season

1. To a food processor, add the cauliflower, yogurt, and olive oil. Process until smooth. 2. Season with salt and pepper before serving.

Per Serving:

calories: 50 | fat: 2g | protein: 4g | carbs: 6g | sugars: 3g | fiber: 3g | sodium: 606mg

Sautéed Spinach and Tomatoes

Prep time: 5 minutes | Cook time: 10 minutes |

Serves 4

1 tablespoon extra-virgin olive
oil
1 cup cherry tomatoes, halved

3 spinach bunches, trimmed
2 garlic cloves, minced
¼ teaspoon salt

1. In a large skillet, heat the oil over medium heat. 2. Add the tomatoes, and cook until the skins begin to blister and split, about 2 minutes. 3. Add the spinach in batches, waiting for each batch to wilt slightly before adding the next batch. Stir continuously for 3 to 4 minutes until the spinach is tender. 4. Add the garlic to the skillet, and toss until fragrant, about 30 seconds. 5. Drain the excess liquid from the pan. Add the salt. Stir well and serve.

Per Serving:

calories: 52 | fat: 4g | protein: 2g | carbs: 4g | sugars: 1g | fiber: 2g | sodium: 183mg

Sherried Peppers with Bean Sprouts

Prep time: 5 minutes | Cook time: 8 minutes | Serves 4

1 green bell pepper, julienned
1 red bell pepper, julienned
2 cups canned, drained bean
sprouts

2 teaspoons light soy sauce
1 tablespoon dry sherry
1 teaspoon red wine vinegar

1. In a large skillet over medium heat, combine the peppers, bean sprouts, soy sauce, and sherry, mixing well. Cover, and cook 5–7 minutes, until the vegetables are just tender. 2. Stir in the vinegar, and remove from the heat. Serve hot.

Per Serving:

calories: 34 | fat: 1g | protein: 2g | carbs: 6g | sugars: 4g | fiber: 2g | sodium: 131mg

Cauliflower with Lime Juice

Prep time: 10 minutes | Cook time: 7 minutes |

Serves 4

2 cups chopped cauliflower
florets
2 tablespoons coconut oil,
melted

2 teaspoons chili powder
½ teaspoon garlic powder
1 medium lime
2 tablespoons chopped cilantro

1. In a large bowl, toss cauliflower with coconut oil. Sprinkle with chili powder and garlic powder. Place seasoned cauliflower into the air fryer basket. 2. Adjust the temperature to 350°F (177°C) and set the timer for 7 minutes. 3. Cauliflower will be tender and begin to turn golden at the edges. Place into a serving bowl. 4. Cut the lime into quarters and squeeze juice over cauliflower. Garnish with cilantro.

Per Serving:

calories: 80 | fat: 7g | protein: 1g | carbs: 5g | fiber: 2g | sodium: 55mg

Roasted Eggplant

Prep time: 15 minutes | Cook time: 15 minutes |

Serves 4

1 large eggplant
2 tablespoons olive oil

¼ teaspoon salt
½ teaspoon garlic powder

1. Remove top and bottom from eggplant. Slice eggplant into ¼-inch-thick round slices. 2. Brush slices with olive oil. Sprinkle with salt and garlic powder. Place eggplant slices into the air fryer basket. 3. Adjust the temperature to 390°F (199°C) and set the timer for 15 minutes. 4. Serve immediately.

Per Serving:

calories: 95| fat: 7g | protein: 1g | carbs: 8g | net carbs: 4g | fiber: 4g

Soft-Baked Tamari Tofu

Prep time: 5 minutes | Cook time: 20 to 25 minutes |
Serves 4

3 tablespoons tamari
1 package (16 ounces) medium-firm tofu

1. Preheat the oven to 425°F. In an ovenproof dish just large enough to hold the tofu, add about half of the tamari. Use several paper towels to pat or squeeze some of the excess moisture from the tofu. Add the tofu to the dish, breaking it up slightly. Sprinkle the remaining tamari over the tofu. Bake for 20 to 25 minutes, or until the tofu is browned and drying in spots. Serve, spooning out tofu with some of the remaining tamari.

Per Serving:
calorie: 87 | fat: 5g | protein: 10g | carbs: 3g | sugars: 1g | fiber: 1g | sodium: 768mg

Pico de Gallo Navy Beans

Prep time: 20 minutes | Cook time: 0 minutes |
Serves 4

2½ cups cooked navy beans
1 tomato, diced
½ red bell pepper, seeded and chopped
¼ jalapeño pepper, chopped
1 scallion, white and green

parts, chopped
1 teaspoon minced garlic
1 teaspoon ground cumin
½ teaspoon ground coriander
½ cup low-sodium feta cheese

1. Put the beans, tomato, bell pepper, jalapeño, scallion, garlic, cumin, and coriander in a medium bowl and stir until well mixed. 2. Top with the feta cheese and serve.

Per Serving:
calories: 218 | fat: 4g | protein: 14g | carbs: 33g | sugars: 2g | fiber: 13g | sodium: 6mg

Brussels Sprouts with Pecans and Gorgonzola

Prep time: 10 minutes | Cook time: 25 minutes |
Serves 4

½ cup pecans
1½ pounds (680 g) fresh Brussels sprouts, trimmed and quartered
2 tablespoons olive oil

Salt and freshly ground black pepper, to taste
¼ cup crumbled Gorgonzola cheese

1. Spread the pecans in a single layer of the air fryer and set the heat to 350ºF (177ºC). Air fry for 3 to 5 minutes until the pecans are lightly browned and fragrant. Transfer the pecans to a plate and continue preheating the air fryer, increasing the heat to 400ºF (204ºC). 2. In a large bowl, toss the Brussels sprouts with the olive oil and season with salt and black pepper to taste. 3. Working in batches if necessary, arrange the Brussels sprouts in a single layer in the air fryer basket. Pausing halfway through the baking time to shake the basket, air fry for 20 to 25 minutes until the sprouts are tender and starting to brown on the edges. 4. Transfer the sprouts to a serving bowl and top with the toasted pecans and Gorgonzola. Serve warm or at room temperature.

Per Serving:
calories: 253 | fat: 18g | protein: 9g | carbs: 17g | fiber: 8g | sodium: 96mg

Lemon-Garlic Mushrooms

Prep time: 10 minutes | Cook time: 10 to 15 minutes
| Serves 6

12 ounces (340 g) sliced mushrooms
1 tablespoon avocado oil
Sea salt and freshly ground black pepper, to taste
3 tablespoons unsalted butter

1 teaspoon minced garlic
1 teaspoon freshly squeezed lemon juice
½ teaspoon red pepper flakes
2 tablespoons chopped fresh parsley

1. Place the mushrooms in a medium bowl and toss with the oil. Season to taste with salt and pepper. 2. Place the mushrooms in a single layer in the air fryer basket. Set your air fryer to 375ºF (191ºC) and roast for 10 to 15 minutes, until the mushrooms are tender. 3. While the mushrooms cook, melt the butter in a small pot or skillet over medium-low heat. Stir in the garlic and cook for 30 seconds. Remove the pot from the heat and stir in the lemon juice and red pepper flakes. 4. Toss the mushrooms with the lemon-garlic butter and garnish with the parsley before serving.

Per Serving:
calories: 72| fat: 6g | protein: 2g | carbs: 3g | net carbs: 2g | fiber: 1g

Horseradish Mashed Cauliflower

Prep time: 5 minutes | Cook time: 10 minutes |
Serves 4

1 large head cauliflower (about 3 pounds), cut into small florets
½ cup skim milk
2 tablespoons prepared

horseradish
¼ teaspoon sea salt
2 teaspoons chopped fresh chives

1. Place a large pot of water on high heat and bring it to a boil. 2. Blanch the cauliflower until it is tender, about 5 minutes. 3. Drain the cauliflower completely and transfer it to a food processor. 4. Add the milk and horseradish to the cauliflower and purée until it is smooth and thick, about 2 minutes. Or mash it by hand with a potato masher. 5. Transfer the mashed cauliflower to a bowl and season with salt. 6. Serve immediately, topped with the chopped chives.

Per Serving:
calories: 102 | fat: 1g | protein: 8g | carbs: 19g | sugars: 9g | fiber: 7g | sodium: 292mg

Garlic Roasted Radishes

Prep time: 5 minutes | Cook time: 15 minutes |

Serves 2 to 4

1 pound radishes, halved
1 tablespoon canola oil
Pinch kosher salt

4 garlic cloves, thinly sliced
¼ cup chopped fresh dill

1. Preheat the oven to 425°F. Line a baking sheet with parchment paper. 2. In a medium bowl, toss the radishes with the canola oil and salt. Spread the vegetables on the prepared baking sheet and roast for 10 minutes. Remove the sheet from the oven, add the garlic, mix well, and return to the oven for 5 minutes. 3. Remove the radishes from the oven, adjust the seasoning as desired, and serve topped with dill on a serving plate or as a side dish. 4. Store any leftovers in an airtight container in the refrigerator for 3 to 4 days.

Per Serving:

calories: 75 | fat: 5g | protein: 1g | carbs: 8g | sugars: 4g | fiber: 3g | sodium: 420mg

Wild Rice Salad with Cranberries and Almonds

Prep time: 10 minutes | Cook time: 25 minutes |

Serves 18

For the rice
2 cups wild rice blend, rinsed
1 teaspoon kosher salt
2½ cups Vegetable Broth or
Chicken Bone Broth
For the dressing
¼ cup extra-virgin olive oil
¼ cup white wine vinegar
1½ teaspoons grated orange zest

Juice of 1 medium orange
(about ¼ cup)
1 teaspoon honey or pure maple syrup
For the salad
¾ cup unsweetened dried cranberries
½ cup sliced almonds, toasted
Freshly ground black pepper

Make the Rice 1. In the electric pressure cooker, combine the rice, salt, and broth. 2. Close and lock the lid. Set the valve to sealing. 3. Cook on high pressure for 25 minutes. 4. When the cooking is complete, hit Cancel and allow the pressure to release naturally for 15 minutes, then quick release any remaining pressure. 5. Once the pin drops, unlock and remove the lid. 6. Let the rice cool briefly, then fluff it with a fork. Make the Dressing 7. While the rice cooks, make the dressing: In a small jar with a screw-top lid, combine the olive oil, vinegar, zest, juice, and honey. (If you don't have a jar, whisk the ingredients together in a small bowl.) Shake to combine. Make the Salad 8. In a large bowl, combine the rice, cranberries, and almonds. 9. Add the dressing and season with pepper. 10. Serve warm or refrigerate.

Per Serving:

calories: 129 | fat: 4g | protein: 3g | carbs: 20g | sugars: 5g | fiber: 2g | sodium: 200mg

Italian Wild Mushrooms

Prep time: 30 minutes | Cook time: 3 minutes |

Serves 10

2 tablespoons canola oil
2 large onions, chopped
4 garlic cloves, minced
3 large red bell peppers, chopped
3 large green bell peppers, chopped
12 ounces package oyster

mushrooms, cleaned and chopped
3 fresh bay leaves
10 fresh basil leaves, chopped
1 teaspoon salt
1½ teaspoons pepper
28 ounces can Italian plum tomatoes, crushed or chopped

1. Press Sauté on the Instant Pot and add in the oil. Once the oil is heated, add the onions, garlic, peppers, and mushroom to the oil. Sauté just until mushrooms begin to turn brown. 2. Add remaining ingredients. Stir well. 3. Secure the lid and make sure vent is set to sealing. Press Manual and set time for 3 minutes. 4. When cook time is up, release the pressure manually. Discard bay leaves.

Per Serving:

calories: 82 | fat: 3g | protein: 3g | carbs: 13g | sugars: 8g | fiber: 4g | sodium: 356mg

Asparagus with Vinaigrette

Prep time: 5 minutes | Cook time: 10 minutes |

Serves 6

1½ pounds fresh or frozen asparagus (thin pieces)
½ cup red wine vinegar
½ teaspoon dried or 1 teaspoon fresh tarragon
2 tablespoons finely chopped fresh chives
3 tablespoons finely chopped fresh parsley

½ cup water
1 tablespoon extra-virgin olive oil
1⅓ tablespoons Dijon mustard
1 pound fresh spinach leaves, trimmed of stems, washed, and dried
2 large tomatoes, cut into wedges

1. Place 1 inch of water in a pot, and place a steamer inside. Arrange the asparagus on top of the steamer. Steam fresh asparagus for 4 minutes or frozen asparagus for 6 to 8 minutes. Immediately rinse the asparagus under cold water to stop the cooking. (This helps keep asparagus bright green and crunchy.) Set aside. 2. In a small bowl or salad cruet, combine the remaining ingredients except the spinach and tomatoes. Mix, or shake well. 3. To serve, line plates with the spinach leaves, and place the asparagus on top of the spinach. Garnish with the tomato wedges, and spoon any remaining dressing on top.

Per Serving:

calories: 72 | fat: 2g | protein: 7g | carbs: 10g | sugars: 2g | fiber: 5g | sodium: 133mg

Caramelized Onions

Prep time: 10 minutes | Cook time: 35 minutes |

Serves 8

4 tablespoons margarine
6 large Vidalia or other sweet onions, sliced into thin half

rings
10 ounces can chicken, or vegetable, broth

1. Press Sauté on the Instant Pot. Add in the margarine and let melt. 2. Once the margarine is melted, stir in the onions and sauté for about 5 minutes. Pour in the broth and then press Cancel. 3. Secure the lid and make sure vent is set to sealing. Press Manual and set time for 20 minutes. 4. When cook time is up, release the pressure manually. Remove the lid and press Sauté. Stir the onion mixture for about 10 more minutes, allowing extra liquid to cook off.

Per Serving:

calorie: 123 | fat: 6g | protein: 2g | carbs: 15g | sugars: 10g | fiber: 3g | sodium: 325mg

Spicy Mustard Greens

Prep time: 10 minutes | Cook time: 15 minutes |

Serves 4

½ cup store-bought low-sodium vegetable broth
½ sweet onion, chopped
1 celery stalk, roughly chopped
½ large red bell pepper, thinly

sliced
2 garlic cloves, minced
1 bunch mustard greens, roughly chopped

1. In a large cast iron pan, bring the broth to a simmer over medium heat. 2. Add the onion, celery, bell pepper, and garlic. Cook, uncovered, stirring occasionally, for 3 to 5 minutes, or until the onion is translucent. 3. Add the mustard greens. Cover the pan, reduce the heat to low, and cook for 10 minutes, or until the greens are wilted. 4. Serve warm.

Per Serving:

calories: 32 | fat: 0g | protein: 1g | carbs: 7g | sugars: 4g | fiber: 2g | sodium: 28mg

Garlic Herb Radishes

Prep time: 10 minutes | Cook time: 10 minutes |

Serves 4

1 pound (454 g) radishes
2 tablespoons unsalted butter, melted
½ teaspoon garlic powder

½ teaspoon dried parsley
¼ teaspoon dried oregano
¼ teaspoon ground black pepper

1. Remove roots from radishes and cut into quarters. 2. In a small

bowl, add butter and seasonings. Toss the radishes in the herb butter and place into the air fryer basket. 3. Adjust the temperature to 350ºF (177ºC) and set the timer for 10 minutes. 4. Halfway through the cooking time, toss the radishes in the air fryer basket. Continue cooking until edges begin to turn brown. 5. Serve warm.

Per Serving:

calories: 57 | fat: 4g | protein: 1g | carbs: 5g | sugars: 3g | fiber: 2g | sodium: 27mg

Teriyaki Chickpeas

Prep time: 5 minutes | Cook time: 20 to 25 minutes |

Serves 7

2 cans (15 ounces each) chickpeas, rinsed and drained
1½ tablespoons tamari
1 tablespoon pure maple syrup

1 tablespoon lemon juice
½ to ¾ teaspoon garlic powder
½ teaspoon ground ginger
½ teaspoon blackstrap molasses

1. Preheat the oven to 450°F. Line a baking sheet with parchment paper. 2. In a large mixing bowl, combine the chickpeas, tamari, syrup, lemon juice, garlic powder, ginger, and molasses. Toss to combine. Spread evenly on the prepared baking sheet and bake for 20 to 25 minutes, or until the marinade is absorbed. Serve warm, or refrigerate to enjoy later.

Per Serving:

calorie: 120 | fat: 2 | protein: 6g | carbs: 20g | sugars: 5g | fiber: 5g | sodium: 382mg

Sun-Dried Tomato Brussels Sprouts

Prep time: 15 minutes | Cook time: 20 minutes |

Serves 4

1 pound Brussels sprouts, trimmed and halved
1 tablespoon extra-virgin olive oil
Sea salt
Freshly ground black pepper

½ cup sun-dried tomatoes, chopped
2 tablespoons freshly squeezed lemon juice
1 teaspoon lemon zest

1. Preheat the oven to 400°F. Line a large baking sheet with aluminum foil. 2. In a large bowl, toss the Brussels sprouts with oil and season with salt and pepper. 3. Spread the Brussels sprouts on the baking sheet in a single layer. 4. Roast the sprouts until they are caramelized, about 20 minutes. 5. Transfer the sprouts to a serving bowl. Mix in the sun-dried tomatoes, lemon juice, and lemon zest. 6. Stir to combine, and serve.

Per Serving:

calories: 98 | fat: 4g | protein: 5g | carbs: 15g | sugars: 5g | fiber: 5g | sodium: 191mg

Kohlrabi Fries

Prep time: 10 minutes | Cook time: 20 to 30 minutes | Serves 4

2 pounds (907 g) kohlrabi, peeled and cut into ¼ to ½-inch fries

2 tablespoons olive oil
Salt and freshly ground black pepper, to taste

1. Preheat the air fryer to 400°F (204°C). 2. In a large bowl, combine the kohlrabi and olive oil. Season to taste with salt and black pepper. Toss gently until thoroughly coated. 3. Working in batches if necessary, spread the kohlrabi in a single layer in the air fryer basket. Pausing halfway through the cooking time to shake the basket, air fry for 20 to 30 minutes until the fries are lightly browned and crunchy.

Per Serving:

calories: 121 | fat: 7g | protein: 4g | carbs: 14g | fiber: 8g | sodium: 45mg

Parmesan-Rosemary Radishes

Prep time: 5 minutes | Cook time: 15 to 20 minutes | Serves 4

1 bunch radishes, stemmed, trimmed, and quartered
1 tablespoon avocado oil
2 tablespoons finely grated fresh Parmesan cheese

1 tablespoon chopped fresh rosemary
Sea salt and freshly ground black pepper, to taste

1. Place the radishes in a medium bowl and toss them with the avocado oil, Parmesan cheese, rosemary, salt, and pepper. 2. Set the air fryer to 375°F (191°C). Arrange the radishes in a single layer in the air fryer basket. Roast for 15 to 20 minutes, until golden brown and tender. Let cool for 5 minutes before serving.

Per Serving:

calories: 58 | fat: 4g | protein: 1g | carbs: 4g | fiber: 2g | sodium: 63mg

Green Beans with Red Peppers

Prep time: 5 minutes | Cook time: 15 minutes | Serves 2

8 ounces fresh green beans, broken into 2-inch pieces
6 sun-dried tomatoes (not packed in oil), halved
1 medium red bell pepper, cut

into ¼-inch strips
1 teaspoon extra-virgin olive oil
Salt, to season
Freshly ground black pepper, to season

1. In a 1-quart saucepan set over high heat, add the green beans to 1 inch of water. Bring to a boil. Boil for 5 minutes, uncovered. 2. Add the sun-dried tomatoes. Cover and boil 5 to 7 minutes more, or until the beans are crisp-tender, and the tomatoes have softened. Drain. Transfer to a serving bowl. 3. Add the red bell pepper and olive oil. Season with salt and pepper. Toss to coat. 4. Serve warm.

Per Serving:

calories: 82 | fat: 3g | protein: 3g | carbs: 13g | sugars: 6g | fiber: 4g | sodium: 601mg

Green Beans with Garlic and Onion

Prep time: 5 minutes | Cook time: 12 minutes | Serves 8

1 pound fresh green beans, trimmed and cut into 2-inch pieces
1 tablespoon extra-virgin olive oil
1 small onion, chopped

1 large garlic clove, minced
1 tablespoon white vinegar
¼ cup Parmigiano-Reggiano cheese
⅛ teaspoon freshly ground black pepper

1. Steam the beans for 7 minutes or until just tender. Set aside. 2. In a skillet, heat the oil over low heat. Add the onion and garlic, and sauté for 4–5 minutes or until the onion is translucent. 3. Transfer the beans to a serving bowl, and add the onion mixture and vinegar, tossing well. Sprinkle with cheese and pepper, and serve.

Per Serving:

calories: 43 | fat: 3g | protein: 1g | carbs: 4g | sugars: 1g | fiber: 1g | sodium: 30mg

Lean Green Avocado Mashed Potatoes

Prep time: 15 minutes | Cook time: 30 minutes | Serves 4

2 large russet potatoes, chopped
1 large head cauliflower, cut into 1-inch (2.5-cm) florets
2 medium leeks, washed and coarsely chopped
2 teaspoons (10 ml) olive oil
1 tablespoon (3 g) dried

rosemary
1 tablespoon (3 g) dried thyme
2 cloves garlic
1 medium avocado, peeled and pitted
2 tablespoons (8 g) finely chopped fresh chives

1. Preheat the oven to 400°F (204°C). 2. Spread out the potatoes, cauliflower, and leeks on a large baking sheet. Drizzle the vegetables with the oil, then sprinkle them with the rosemary and thyme. Add the garlic to the baking sheet. Bake the vegetables for about 30 minutes, until the potatoes are fork-tender. 3. Transfer the vegetables to a food processor and add the avocado. Process the mixture to the desired consistency. 4. Top the mashed potatoes with the chives and serve.

Per Serving:

calorie: 248 | fat: 10g | protein: 7g | carbs: 37g | sugars: 6g | fiber: 9g | sodium: 69mg

Garlicky Cabbage and Collard Greens

Prep time: 10 minutes | Cook time: 10 minutes |

Serves 8

2 tablespoons extra-virgin olive oil
1 collard greens bunch, stemmed and thinly sliced
½ small green cabbage, thinly sliced
6 garlic cloves, minced
1 tablespoon low-sodium gluten-free soy sauce or tamari

1. In a large skillet, heat the oil over medium-high heat. 2. Add the collards to the pan, stirring to coat with oil. Sauté for 1 to 2 minutes until the greens begin to wilt. 3. Add the cabbage and stir to coat. Cover and reduce the heat to medium low. Continue to cook for 5 to 7 minutes, stirring once or twice, until the greens are tender. 4. Add the garlic and soy sauce and stir to incorporate. Cook until just fragrant, about 30 seconds longer. Serve warm and enjoy!

Per Serving:
calories: 72| fat: 4g | protein: 3g | carbs: 6g | sugars: 0g | fiber: 3g | sodium: 129mg

Moreish Lemony Quinoa

Prep time: 5 minutes | Cook time: 15 minutes |

Serves 3

1 cup dry quinoa, rinsed and drained
1¾ cups water
2½ tablespoons tamari
2 tablespoons tahini
3 to 4 tablespoons fresh lemon juice
½ teaspoon garlic powder

1. In a large saucepan over high heat, combine the quinoa and water. Bring to a boil, stir, then reduce the heat to low. Cover and cook for 11 minutes. In a small bowl, combine the tamari, tahini, lemon juice, and garlic powder. Whisk to combine. Once the quinoa is cooked, turn off the heat and stir in the tahini mixture. Cover again, let sit for a couple of minutes, and serve.

Per Serving:
calorie: 281 | fat: 9g | protein: 11g | carbs: 40g | sugars: 4g | fiber: 5g | sodium: 861mg

Broiled Asparagus

Prep time: 5 minutes | Cook time: 5 to 6 minutes |

Serves 3

1 pound asparagus
1 teaspoon lemon juice
¼ teaspoon sea salt
Lemon pepper (optional)

1. Set the oven or toaster oven to broil. Line a baking sheet with parchment paper. 2. Wash and trim the asparagus. (Use a knife or break off ends where they naturally snap.) Pat the asparagus dry, and transfer to the prepared baking sheet. Sprinkle with the lemon juice, toss to coat, and then sprinkle with the salt. Broil for 5 to 6 minutes, or until the asparagus turns bright green. Remove, sprinkle with the lemon pepper (if using), and serve.

Per Serving:
calorie: 17 | fat: 0g | protein: 2g | carbs: 3g | sugars: 1g | fiber: 2g | sodium: 206mg

Zucchini Ribbons with Tarragon

Prep time: 5 minutes | Cook time: 1 minutes | Serves 2

1 zucchini, thinly sliced lengthwise into ribbons
1 tablespoon nonfat ricotta cheese
1 tablespoon pine nuts
1 tablespoon fresh tarragon
1½ teaspoons extra-virgin olive oil
½ to 1 teaspoon red pepper flakes

1. Bring a large pot of water to a boil. 2. Add the zucchini. Cook for 30 to 60 seconds, or until crisp-tender. Drain. Transfer the zucchini to a serving bowl. 3. Add the ricotta cheese, pine nuts, tarragon, olive oil, and red pepper flakes. Gently toss until the zucchini is coated. 4. Serve and enjoy!

Per Serving:
calories: 62 | fat: 5g | protein: 2g | carbs: 3g | sugars: 1g | fiber: 1g | sodium: 15mg

Artichokes Parmesan

Prep time: 5 minutes | Cook time: 20 minutes |

Serves 6

½ cup dried whole-wheat bread crumbs
2 tablespoons grated Parmigiano-Reggiano cheese
⅛ teaspoon freshly ground black pepper
9 ounces frozen artichoke hearts, thawed
2 tablespoons extra-virgin olive oil, divided
2 medium tomatoes, diced

1. Preheat the oven to 425 degrees. 2. In a small bowl, combine the bread crumbs, cheese, and black pepper, and stir to combine. 3. Arrange the artichoke hearts in a 1-quart casserole dish. Sprinkle the tomatoes over the top. Season with salt, if desired. 4. Sprinkle the bread crumb mixture over the vegetables, and bake for 15 to 20 minutes or until the topping is light brown.

Per Serving:
calories: 78 | fat: 5g | protein: 2g | carbs:7 g | sugars: 1g | fiber: 2g | sodium: 67mg

Garlic Roasted Broccoli

Prep time: 8 minutes | Cook time: 10 to 14 minutes | Serves 6

1 head broccoli, cut into bite-size florets
1 tablespoon avocado oil
2 teaspoons minced garlic
⅛ teaspoon red pepper flakes

Sea salt and freshly ground black pepper, to taste
1 tablespoon freshly squeezed lemon juice
½ teaspoon lemon zest

1. In a large bowl, toss together the broccoli, avocado oil, garlic, red pepper flakes, salt, and pepper. 2. Set the air fryer to 375°F (191°C). Arrange the broccoli in a single layer in the air fryer basket, working in batches if necessary. Roast for 10 to 14 minutes, until the broccoli is lightly charred. 3. Place the florets in a medium bowl and toss with the lemon juice and lemon zest. Serve.

Per Serving:
calories: 58 | fat: 3g | protein: 3g | carbs: 7g | fiber: 3g | sodium: 34mg

Sweet-and-Sour Cabbage Slaw

Prep time: 10 minutes | Cook time: 0 minutes | Serves 2

2 tablespoons apple cider vinegar
1 tablespoon granulated stevia
2 cups angel hair cabbage
1 tart apple, cored and diced

½ cup shredded carrot
2 medium scallions, sliced
2 tablespoons sliced almonds

1. In a medium bowl, stir together the vinegar and stevia. 2. In a large bowl, mix together the cabbage, apple, carrot, and scallions. 3. Pour the sweetened vinegar over the vegetable mixture. Toss to combine. 4. Garnish with the sliced almonds and serve.

Per Serving:
calories: 125 | fat: 1g | protein: 2g | carbs: 30g | sugars: 21g | fiber: 5g | sodium: 47mg

Chapter 9 Vegetarian Mains

Crispy Eggplant Rounds

Prep time: 15 minutes | Cook time: 10 minutes |
Serves 4

1 large eggplant, ends trimmed, cut into ½-inch slices
½ teaspoon salt
2 ounces (57 g) Parmesan 100%
cheese crisps, finely ground
½ teaspoon paprika
¼ teaspoon garlic powder
1 large egg

1. Sprinkle eggplant rounds with salt. Place rounds on a kitchen towel for 30 minutes to draw out excess water. Pat rounds dry. 2. In a medium bowl, mix cheese crisps, paprika, and garlic powder. In a separate medium bowl, whisk egg. Dip each eggplant round in egg, then gently press into cheese crisps to coat both sides. 3. Place eggplant rounds into ungreased air fryer basket. Adjust the temperature to 400°F (204°C) and air fry for 10 minutes, turning rounds halfway through cooking. Eggplant will be golden and crispy when done. Serve warm.

Per Serving:
calories: 113 | fat: 5g | protein: 7g | carbs: 10g | fiber: 4g | sodium: 567mg

Stuffed Acorn Squash

Prep time: 10 minutes | Cook time: 1 hour | Serves 2

1 acorn squash, halved and seeded
½ cup water, plus more as needed
¼ cup uncooked quinoa, thoroughly rinsed
1 tablespoon extra-virgin olive oil
¼ cup diced onion
1 garlic clove, chopped
½ cup broccoli florets
½ cup frozen peas
Salt, to season
Freshly ground black pepper, to season
4 tablespoons chopped pistachios, divided

1. Preheat the oven to 425°F. 2. In a large baking dish, place the acorn squash halves cut-side down. Add 1 inch of water to the dish. Place the dish in the preheated oven. Bake for 45 minutes, or until tender. 3. In a small pot set over high heat, bring the water to a boil. 4. Add the quinoa. Reduce the heat to low. Simmer for about 15 minutes, covered, or until tender and all the water is absorbed. Let cool. Fluff with a fork. 5. In a medium saucepan set over medium heat, add the olive oil, onion, and garlic. Sauté for 3 to 4 minutes. 6. Add the broccoli and peas. Cook for about 4 minutes, or until the vegetables are tender. 7. Add the cooked quinoa to the sautéed vegetables. Season with salt and pepper. 8. Spoon half of the mixture into each acorn half. 9. Garnish each half with about 2 tablespoons of pistachios. 10. Serve hot and enjoy!

Per Serving:
calories: 306 | fat: 12g | protein: 10g | carbs: 46g | sugars: 2g | fiber: 8g | sodium: 656mg

Italian Zucchini Boats

Prep time: 5 minutes | Cook time: 15 minutes |
Serves 4

1 cup canned low-sodium chickpeas, drained and rinsed
1 cup no-sugar-added spaghetti sauce
2 zucchini
¼ cup shredded Parmesan cheese

1. Preheat the oven to 425°F. 2. In a medium bowl, mix the chickpeas and spaghetti sauce together. 3. Cut the zucchini in half lengthwise, and scrape a spoon gently down the length of each half to remove the seeds. 4. Fill each zucchini half with the chickpea sauce, and top with one-quarter of the Parmesan cheese. 5. Place the zucchini halves on a baking sheet and roast in the oven for 15 minutes.

Per Serving:
calories: 120 | fat: 4g | protein: 7g | carbs: 14g | sugars: 5g | fiber: 4g | sodium: 441mg

Roasted Veggie Bowl

Prep time: 10 minutes | Cook time: 15 minutes |
Serves 2

1 cup broccoli florets
1 cup quartered Brussels sprouts
½ cup cauliflower florets
¼ medium white onion, peeled and sliced ¼ inch thick
½ medium green bell pepper, seeded and sliced ¼ inch thick
1 tablespoon coconut oil
2 teaspoons chili powder
½ teaspoon garlic powder
½ teaspoon cumin

1. Toss all ingredients together in a large bowl until vegetables are fully coated with oil and seasoning. 2. Pour vegetables into the air fryer basket. 3. Adjust the temperature to 360°F (182°C) and roast for 15 minutes. 4. Shake two or three times during cooking. Serve warm.

Per Serving:
calories: 112 | fat: 8g | protein: 4g | carbs: 11g | sugars: 3g | fiber: 5g | sodium: 106mg

No-Bake Spaghetti Squash Casserole

Prep time: 10 minutes | Cook time: 45 minutes |

Serves 6

Marinara
3 tablespoons extra-virgin olive oil
3 garlic cloves, minced
One 28-ounce can whole San Marzano tomatoes and their liquid
2 teaspoons Italian seasoning
1 teaspoon fine sea salt
½ teaspoon red pepper flakes (optional)
Vegan Parmesan
½ cup raw whole cashews
2 tablespoons nutritional yeast
½ teaspoon garlic powder
½ teaspoon fine sea salt
Vegan Ricotta
One 14-ounce package firm tofu, drained
½ cup raw whole cashews,
soaked in water to cover for 1 to 2 hours and then drained
3 tablespoons nutritional yeast
2 tablespoons extra-virgin olive oil
1 teaspoon finely grated lemon zest, plus 2 tablespoons fresh lemon juice
½ cup firmly packed fresh flat-leaf parsley leaves
1½ teaspoons Italian seasoning
1 teaspoon garlic powder
1 teaspoon fine sea salt
½ teaspoon freshly ground black pepper
One 3½-pound steamed spaghetti squash
2 tablespoons chopped fresh flat-leaf parsley

1. To make the marinara: Select the Sauté setting on the Instant Pot and heat the oil and garlic for about 2 minutes, until the garlic is bubbling but not browned. Add the tomatoes and their liquid and use a wooden spoon or spatula to crush the tomatoes against the side of the pot. Stir in the Italian seasoning, salt, and pepper flakes (if using) and cook, stirring occasionally, for about 10 minutes, until the sauce has thickened a bit. Press the Cancel button to turn off the pot and let the sauce cook from the residual heat for about 5 minutes more, until it is no longer simmering. Wearing heat-resistant mitts, lift the pot out of the housing, pour the sauce into a medium heatproof bowl, and set aside. (You can make the sauce up to 4 days in advance, then let it cool, transfer it to an airtight container, and refrigerate.) 2. To make the vegan Parmesan: In a food processor, combine the cashews, nutritional yeast, garlic powder, and salt. Using 1-second pulses, pulse about ten times, until the mixture resembles grated Parmesan cheese. Transfer to a small bowl and set aside. Do not wash the food processor bowl and blade. 3. To make the vegan ricotta: Cut the tofu crosswise into eight ½-inch-thick slices. Sandwich the slices between double layers of paper towels or a folded kitchen towel and press gently to remove excess moisture. Add the tofu to the food processor along with the cashews, nutritional yeast, oil, lemon zest, lemon juice, parsley, Italian seasoning, garlic powder, salt, and pepper. Process for about 1 minute, until the mixture is mostly smooth with flecks of parsley throughout. Set aside. 4. Return the marinara to the pot. Select the Sauté setting and heat the marinara sauce for about 3 minutes, until it starts to simmer. Add the spaghetti squash and vegan ricotta to the pot and stir to combine. Continue to heat, stirring often, for 8 to 10 minutes, until piping hot. Press the Cancel button to turn off the pot. 5. Spoon the spaghetti squash into bowls, top with the vegan Parmesan and parsley, and serve right away.

Per Serving:

calorie: 307 | fat: 17g | protein: 16g | carbs: 25g | sugars: 2g | fiber: 5g | sodium: 985mg

Sautéed Spinach and Lima Beans

Prep time: 5 minutes | Cook time: 40 minutes |

Serves 2

Extra-virgin olive oil cooking spray
¼ cup chopped onion
½ cup low-sodium vegetable broth
1 cup frozen lima beans, thawed
2 teaspoons extra-virgin olive oil
2 garlic cloves, chopped
4 cups chopped fresh spinach
Pinch cayenne pepper
2 teaspoons balsamic vinegar
Salt, to season
Freshly ground black pepper, to season

1. Heat a large saucepan over medium heat. Spray with cooking spray. 2. Add the onion. Sauté for about 4 minutes, or until soft and translucent. 3. Add the vegetable broth. Bring to a boil. 4. Add the lima beans and just enough water to cover. Bring to a boil. Reduce the heat to low. Cover and simmer for 30 minutes, or until the beans are tender. Set aside. 5. Heat a large skillet over medium-high heat for 30 seconds. 6. Add the olive oil and garlic. Sauté for 1 to 2 minutes, or until golden. Remove the garlic and reserve. 7. To the skillet, add the spinach and cayenne. Cover and cook for about 1 minute, or until the leaves wilt. Drain to remove any excess water. 8. Stir in the balsamic vinegar. Season with salt and pepper. 9. To serve, mound half of the spinach on a plate, top with half of the lima beans, and sprinkle with the reserved garlic.

Per Serving:

calories: 201 | fat: 7g | protein: 9g | carbs: 29g | sugars: 3g | fiber: 7g | sodium: 418mg

Orange Tofu

Prep time: 10 minutes | Cook time: 20 minutes |

Serves 4

⅓ cup freshly squeezed orange juice (zest orange first; see orange zest ingredient below)
1 tablespoon tamari
1 tablespoon tahini
½ tablespoon coconut nectar or pure maple syrup
2 tablespoons apple cider vinegar
½ tablespoon freshly grated
ginger
1 large clove garlic, grated
½ to 1 teaspoon orange zest
¼ teaspoon sea salt
Few pinches of crushed red-pepper flakes (optional)
1 package (12 ounces) extra-firm tofu, sliced into ¼"–½" thick squares and patted to remove excess moisture

1. Preheat the oven to 400°F. 2. In a small bowl, combine the orange juice, tamari, tahini, nectar or syrup, vinegar, ginger, garlic, orange zest, salt, and red-pepper flakes (if using). Whisk until well combined. Pour the sauce into an 8" x 12" baking dish. Add the tofu and turn to coat both sides. Bake for 20 minutes. Add salt to taste.

Per Serving:

calorie: 122 | fat: 7g | protein: 10g | carbs: 7g | sugars: 4g | fiber: 1g | sodium: 410mg

Crispy Cabbage Steaks

Prep time: 5 minutes | Cook time: 10 minutes |
Serves 4

1 small head green cabbage, cored and cut into ½-inch-thick slices	2 tablespoons olive oil
¼ teaspoon salt	1 clove garlic, peeled and finely minced
¼ teaspoon ground black pepper	½ teaspoon dried thyme
	½ teaspoon dried parsley

1. Sprinkle each side of cabbage with salt and pepper, then place into ungreased air fryer basket, working in batches if needed. 2. Drizzle each side of cabbage with olive oil, then sprinkle with remaining ingredients on both sides. Adjust the temperature to 350°F (177°C) and air fry for 10 minutes, turning "steaks" halfway through cooking. 3.Cabbage will be browned at the edges and tender when done. Serve warm.

Per Serving:

calories: 63 | fat: 7g | protein: 0g | carbs: 1g | fiber: 0g | sodium: 155mg

Chile Relleno Casserole with Salsa Salad

Prep time: 10 minutes | Cook time: 55 minutes |
Serves 4

Casserole	2 Roma tomatoes, seeded and diced
½ cup gluten-free flour (such as King Arthur)	1 green bell pepper, seeded and diced
1 teaspoon baking powder	½ small yellow onion, diced
6 large eggs	1 jalapeño chile, seeded and diced (optional)
½ cup nondairy milk or whole milk	2 tablespoons chopped fresh cilantro
Three 4 ounces cans fire-roasted diced green chiles, drained	4 teaspoons extra-virgin olive oil
1 cup nondairy cheese shreds or shredded mozzarella cheese	4 teaspoons fresh lime juice
Salad	⅛ teaspoon fine sea salt
1 head green leaf lettuce, shredded	

1. To make the casserole: Pour 1 cup water into the Instant Pot. Butter a 7-cup round heatproof glass dish or coat with nonstick cooking spray and place the dish on a long-handled silicone steam rack. (If you don't have the long-handled rack, use the wire metal steam rack and a homemade sling) 2. In a medium bowl, whisk together the flour and baking powder. Add the eggs and milk and whisk until well blended, forming a batter. Stir in the chiles and ¾ cup of the cheese. 3. Pour the batter into the prepared dish and cover tightly with aluminum foil. Holding the handles of the steam rack, lower the dish into the Instant Pot. 4. Secure the lid and set the Pressure Release to Sealing. Select the Pressure Cook or Manual setting and set the cooking time for 40 minutes at high pressure. (The pot will take about 10 minutes to come up to pressure before

the cooking program begins.) 5. When the cooking program ends, let the pressure release naturally for at least 10 minutes, then move the Pressure Release to Venting to release any remaining steam. Open the pot and, wearing heat-resistant mitts, grasp the handles of the steam rack and lift it out of the pot. Uncover the dish, taking care not to get burned by the steam or to drip condensation onto the casserole. While the casserole is still piping hot, sprinkle the remaining ¼ cup cheese evenly on top. Let the cheese melt for 5 minutes. 6. To make the salad: While the cheese is melting, in a large bowl, combine the lettuce, tomatoes, bell pepper, onion, jalapeño (if using), cilantro, oil, lime juice, and salt. Toss until evenly combined. 7. Cut the casserole into wedges. Serve warm, with the salad on the side.

Per Serving:

calorie: 361 | fat: 22g | protein: 21g | carbs: 23g | sugars: 8g | fiber: 3g | sodium: 421mg

Gingered Tofu and Greens

Prep time: 15 minutes | Cook time: 20 minutes |
Serves 2

For the marinade	oil, divided
2 tablespoons low-sodium soy sauce	1 tablespoon grated fresh ginger
¼ cup rice vinegar	2 cups coarsely shredded bok choy
⅓ cup water	2 cups coarsely shredded kale, thoroughly washed
1 tablespoon grated fresh ginger	½ cup fresh, or frozen, chopped green beans
1 tablespoon coconut flour	
1 teaspoon granulated stevia	1 tablespoon freshly squeezed lime juice
1 garlic clove, minced	
For the tofu and greens	1 tablespoon chopped fresh cilantro
8 ounces extra-firm tofu, drained, cut into 1-inch cubes	
3 teaspoons extra-virgin olive	2 tablespoons hemp hearts

To make the marinade 1. In a small bowl, whisk together the soy sauce, rice vinegar, water, ginger, coconut flour, stevia, and garlic until well combined. 2. Place a small saucepan set over high heat. Add the marinade. Bring to a boil. Cook for 1 minute. Remove from the heat. To make the tofu and greens 1. In a medium ovenproof pan, place the tofu in a single layer. Pour the marinade over. Drizzle with 1½ teaspoons of olive oil. Let sit for 5 minutes. 2. Preheat the broiler to high. 3. Place the pan under the broiler. Broil the tofu for 7 to 8 minutes, or until lightly browned. Using a spatula, turn the tofu over. Continue to broil for 7 to 8 minutes more, or until browned on this side. 4. In a large wok or skillet set over high heat, heat the remaining 1½ teaspoons of olive oil. 5. Stir in the ginger. 6. Add the bok choy, kale, and green beans. Cook for 2 to 3 minutes, stirring constantly, until the greens wilt. 7. Add the lime juice and cilantro. Remove from the heat. 8. Add the browned tofu with any remaining marinade in the pan to the bok choy, kale, and green beans. Toss gently to combine. 9. Top with the hemp hearts and serve immediately.

Per Serving:

calories: 252 | fat: 14g | protein: 15g | carbs: 20g | sugars: 4g | fiber: 3g | sodium: 679mg

Cheesy Zucchini Patties

Prep time: 10 minutes | Cook time: 20 minutes |

Serves 2

1 cup grated zucchini
1 cup chopped fresh mushrooms
½ cup grated carrot
½ cup nonfat shredded mozzarella cheese
¼ cup finely ground flaxseed
1 large egg, beaten
1 garlic clove, minced

Salt, to season
Freshly ground black pepper, to season
1 tablespoon extra-virgin olive oil
4 cup mixed baby greens, divided

1. In a medium bowl, stir together the zucchini, mushrooms, carrot, mozzarella cheese, flaxseed, egg, and garlic. Season with salt and pepper. Stir again to combine. 2. In a large skillet set over medium-high heat, heat the olive oil. 3. Drop 1 tablespoon of the zucchini mixture into the skillet. Continue dropping tablespoon-size portions in the pan until it is full, but not crowded. Cook for 2 to 3 minutes on each side, or until golden. Transfer to a serving plate. Repeat with the remaining mixture. 4. Place 2 cups of greens on each serving plate. Top each with zucchini patties. 5. Enjoy!

Per Serving:
calories: 252 | fat: 15g | protein: 19g | carbs: 14g | sugars: 4g | fiber: 9g | sodium: 644mg

Edamame Falafel with Roasted Vegetables

Prep time: 10 minutes | Cook time: 55 minutes |

Serves 2

For the roasted vegetables
1 cup broccoli florets
1 medium zucchini, sliced
½ cup cherry tomatoes, halved
1½ teaspoons extra-virgin olive oil
Salt, to season
Freshly ground black pepper, to season
Extra-virgin olive oil cooking spray
For the falafel
1 cup frozen shelled edamame, thawed

1 small onion, chopped
1 garlic clove, chopped
1 tablespoon freshly squeezed lemon juice
2 tablespoons hemp hearts
1 teaspoon ground cumin
2 tablespoons oat flour
¼ teaspoon salt
Pinch freshly ground black pepper
2 tablespoons extra-virgin olive oil, divided
Prepared hummus, for serving (optional)

To make the roasted vegetables 1. Preheat the oven to 425°F. 2. In a large bowl, toss together the broccoli, zucchini, tomatoes, and olive oil to coat. Season with salt and pepper. 3. Spray a baking sheet with cooking spray. 4. Spread the vegetables evenly atop the sheet. Place the sheet in the preheated oven. Roast for 35 to 40 minutes, stirring every 15 minutes, or until the vegetables are soft and cooked through. 5. Remove from the oven. Set aside. To make the falafel 1. In a food processor, pulse the edamame until coarsely ground. 2. Add the onion, garlic, lemon juice, and hemp hearts.

Process until finely ground. Transfer the mixture to a medium bowl. 3. By hand, mix in the cumin, oat flour, salt, and pepper. 4. Roll the dough into 1-inch balls. Flatten slightly. You should have about 12 silver dollar–size patties. 5. In a large skillet set over medium heat, heat 1 tablespoon of olive oil. 6. Add 4 falafel patties to the pan at a time (or as many as will fit without crowding), and cook for about 3 minutes on each side, or until lightly browned. Remove from the pan. Repeat with the remaining 1 tablespoon of olive oil and falafel patties. 7. Serve immediately with the roasted vegetables and hummus (if using) and enjoy!

Per Serving:
calories: 316 | fat: 22g | protein: 12g | carbs: 21g | sugars: 4g | fiber: 6g | sodium: 649mg

Parmesan Artichokes

Prep time: 10 minutes | Cook time: 10 minutes |

Serves 4

2 medium artichokes, trimmed and quartered, center removed
2 tablespoons coconut oil
1 large egg, beaten
½ cup grated vegetarian

Parmesan cheese
¼ cup blanched finely ground almond flour
½ teaspoon crushed red pepper flakes

1. In a large bowl, toss artichokes in coconut oil and then dip each piece into the egg. 2. Mix the Parmesan and almond flour in a large bowl. Add artichoke pieces and toss to cover as completely as possible, sprinkle with pepper flakes. Place into the air fryer basket. 3. Adjust the temperature to 400°F (204°C) and air fry for 10 minutes. 4. Toss the basket two times during cooking. Serve warm.

Per Serving:
calories: 207 | fat: 13g | protein: 10g | carbs: 15g | fiber: 5g | sodium: 211mg

No-Tuna Lettuce Wraps

Prep time: 10 minutes | Cook time: 0 minutes |

Serves 4

1 (15 ounces) can low-sodium chickpeas, drained and rinsed
1 celery stalk, thinly sliced
3 tablespoons honey mustard
2 tablespoons finely chopped

red onion
2 tablespoons unsalted tahini
1 tablespoon capers, undrained
12 butter lettuce leaves

1. In a large bowl, mash the chickpeas. 2. Add the celery, honey mustard, onion, tahini, and capers, and mix well. 3. For each serving, place three lettuce leaves on a plate so they overlap, top with one-fourth of the chickpea filling, and roll up into a wrap. Repeat with the remaining lettuce leaves and filling.

Per Serving:
calories: 163 | fat: 8g | protein: 6g | carbs: 17g | sugars: 4g | fiber: 6g | sodium: 333mg

Tofu and Bean Chili

Prep time: 10 minutes | Cook time 30 minutes |
Serves 4

1 (15 ounces) can low-sodium dark red kidney beans, drained and rinsed, divided	½ teaspoon chili powder
	½ teaspoon ground cumin
	½ teaspoon garlic powder
2 (15 ounces) cans no-salt-added diced tomatoes	½ teaspoon dried oregano
	¼ teaspoon onion powder
1½ cups low-sodium vegetable broth	¼ teaspoon salt
	8 ounces extra-firm tofu

1. In a small bowl, mash ⅓ of the beans with a fork. 2. Put the mashed beans, the remaining whole beans, and the diced tomatoes with their juices in a large stockpot. 3. Add the broth, chili powder, cumin, garlic powder, dried oregano, onion powder, and salt. Simmer over medium-high heat for 15 minutes. 4. Press the tofu between 3 or 4 layers of paper towels to squeeze out any excess moisture. 5. Crumble the tofu into the stockpot and stir. Simmer for another 10 to 15 minutes.

Per Serving:

calories: 207 | fat: 5g | protein: 15g | carbs: 31g | sugars: 11g | fiber: 12g | sodium: 376mg

Vegan Dal Makhani

Prep time: 0 minutes | Cook time: 55 minutes |
Serves 6

1 cup dried kidney beans	diced
⅓ cup urad dal or beluga or Puy lentils	1 tablespoon garam masala
	1 teaspoon ground turmeric
4 cups water	¼ teaspoon cayenne pepper (optional)
1 teaspoon fine sea salt	
1 tablespoon cold-pressed avocado oil	One 15 ounces can fire-roasted diced tomatoes and liquid
1 tablespoon cumin seeds	2 tablespoons vegan buttery spread
1-inch piece fresh ginger, peeled and minced	Cooked cauliflower "rice" for serving
4 garlic cloves, minced	
1 large yellow onion, diced	2 tablespoons chopped fresh cilantro
2 jalapeño chiles, seeded and diced	
1 green bell pepper, seeded and	6 tablespoons plain coconut yogurt

1. In a medium bowl, combine the kidney beans, urad dal, water, and salt and stir to dissolve the salt. Let soak for 12 hours. 2. Select the Sauté setting on the Instant Pot and heat the oil and cumin seeds for 3 minutes, until the seeds are bubbling, lightly toasted, and aromatic. Add the ginger and garlic and sauté for 1 minute, until bubbling and fragrant. Add the onion, jalapeños, and bell pepper and sauté for 5 minutes, until the onion begins to soften. 3. Add the garam masala, turmeric, cayenne (if using), and the soaked beans and their liquid and stir to mix. Pour the tomatoes and their liquid on top. Do not stir them in. 4. Secure the lid and set the Pressure Release to Sealing. Press the Cancel button to reset the cooking program, then select the Pressure Cook or Manual setting and set the cooking time for 30 minutes at high pressure. (The pot will

take about 15 minutes to come up to pressure before the cooking program begins.) 5. When the cooking program ends, let the pressure release naturally for 30 minutes, then move the Pressure Release to Venting to release any remaining steam. Open the pot and stir to combine, then stir in the buttery spread. If you prefer a smoother texture, ladle 1½ cups of the dal into a blender and blend until smooth, about 30 seconds, then stir the blended mixture into the rest of the dal in the pot. 6. Spoon the cauliflower "rice" into bowls and ladle the dal on top. Sprinkle with the cilantro, top with a dollop of coconut yogurt, and serve.

Per Serving:

calorie: 245 | fat: 7g | protein: 11g | carbs: 37g | sugars: 4g | fiber: 10g | sodium: 518mg

Mushroom and Cauliflower Rice Risotto

Prep time: 5 minutes | Cook time: 10 minutes |
Serves 4

1 teaspoon extra-virgin olive oil	broth
½ cup chopped portobello mushrooms	½ cup half-and-half
	1 cup shredded Parmesan cheese
4 cups cauliflower rice	
¼ cup low-sodium vegetable	

1. Heat the oil in a medium skillet over medium-low heat. When hot, put the mushrooms in the skillet and cook for 3 minutes, stirring once. 2. Add the cauliflower rice, broth, and half-and-half. Stir and cover. Increase to high heat and boil for 5 minutes. 3. Add the cheese. Stir to incorporate. Cook for 3 more minutes.

Per Serving:

calories: 159 | fat: 8g | protein: 10g | carbs: 12g | sugars: 4g | fiber: 2g | sodium: 531mg

Chickpea Coconut Curry

Prep time: 5 minutes | Cook time: 15 minutes |
Serves 4

3 cups fresh or frozen cauliflower florets	chickpeas, drained and rinsed
	1 tablespoon curry powder
2 cups unsweetened almond milk	¼ teaspoon ground ginger
	¼ teaspoon garlic powder
1 (15 ounces) can coconut milk	⅛ teaspoon onion powder
1 (15 ounces) can low-sodium	¼ teaspoon salt

1. In a large stockpot, combine the cauliflower, almond milk, coconut milk, chickpeas, curry, ginger, garlic powder, and onion powder. Stir and cover. 2. Cook over medium-high heat for 10 minutes. 3. Reduce the heat to low, stir, and cook for 5 minutes more, uncovered. Season with up to ¼ teaspoon salt.

Per Serving:

calories: 225 | fat: 7g | protein: 12g | carbs: 31g | sugars: 14g | fiber: 9g | sodium: 489mg

Easy Cheesy Vegetable Frittata

Prep time: 10 minutes | Cook time: 15 minutes |

Serves 2

Extra-virgin olive oil cooking spray	basil
½ cup sliced onion	Pinch freshly ground black pepper
½ cup sliced green bell pepper	½ cup liquid egg substitute
½ cup sliced eggplant	½ cup nonfat cottage cheese
½ cup frozen spinach	¼ cup fat-free evaporated milk
½ cup sliced fresh mushrooms	¼ cup nonfat shredded Cheddar cheese
1 tablespoon chopped fresh	

1. Coat an ovenproof 10-inch skillet with cooking spray. Place it over medium-low heat until hot. 2. Add the onion, green bell pepper, eggplant, spinach, and mushrooms. Sauté for 2 to 3 minutes, or until lightly browned. 3. Add the basil. Season with pepper. Stir to combine. Cook for 2 to 3 minutes more, or until the flavors blend. Remove from the heat. 4. Preheat the broiler. 5. In a blender, combine the egg substitute, cottage cheese, Cheddar cheese, and evaporated milk. Process until smooth. Pour the egg mixture over the vegetables in the skillet. 6. Return the skillet to medium-low heat. Cover and cook for about 5 minutes, or until the bottom sets and the top is still slightly wet. 7. Transfer the ovenproof skillet to the broiler. Broil for 2 to 3 minutes, or until the top is set. 8. Serve one-half of the frittata per person and enjoy!

Per Serving:

calories: 177 | fat: 7g | protein: 17g | carbs: 12g | sugars: 6g | fiber: 3g | sodium: 408mg

Stuffed Peppers

Prep time: 20 minutes | Cook time: 50 minutes |

Serves 2

½ cup water	Salt, to season
¼ cup uncooked quinoa, thoroughly rinsed	Freshly ground black pepper, to season
1 tablespoon extra-virgin olive oil	1 red bell pepper, halved and seeded
1 garlic clove, minced	1 orange bell pepper, halved and seeded
6 ounces extra-firm tofu, drained and sliced	½ cup nonfat shredded mozzarella cheese, divided
½ cup marinara sauce, divided	4 tomato slices, divided
¼ cup finely chopped walnuts	
1 teaspoon dried basil	

1. Preheat the oven to 350°F. 2. In a small pot set over high heat, bring the water to a boil. 3. Add the quinoa. Reduce the heat to low. Cover and simmer for about 15 minutes, or until tender and all the water is absorbed. Let cool. Fluff with a fork. Set aside. 4. In a skillet set over medium heat, stir together the olive oil, garlic, and tofu. Cook for about 5 minutes, or until the tofu is evenly brown. 5. Mix in ¼ cup of marinara, the walnuts, and basil. Season with salt and pepper. Cook for 5 minutes more, stirring. 6. Using a wooden spoon or spatula, press one-quarter of the cooked quinoa into each pepper half. 7. Top each with about 1 tablespoon of the remaining ¼ cup of marinara. 8. Sprinkle each with about 1 tablespoon of mozzarella cheese. 9. Place 1 tomato slice on each filled pepper. 10. Finish with about 1 tablespoon of the remaining ¼ cup of mozzarella cheese. 11. Transfer the stuffed peppers to a baking dish. Place the dish in the preheated oven. Bake for 25 minutes, or until the cheese melts. 12. Serve 1 stuffed red bell pepper half and 1 stuffed orange bell pepper half to each person and enjoy!

Per Serving:

calories: 399 | fat: 21g | protein: 25g | carbs: 33g | sugars: 7g | fiber: 6g | sodium: 535mg

Stuffed Portobellos

Prep time: 10 minutes | Cook time: 8 minutes |

Serves 4

3 ounces (85 g) cream cheese, softened	leaves
½ medium zucchini, trimmed and chopped	4 large portobello mushrooms, stems removed
¼ cup seeded and chopped red bell pepper	2 tablespoons coconut oil, melted
1½ cups chopped fresh spinach	½ teaspoon salt

1. In a medium bowl, mix cream cheese, zucchini, pepper, and spinach. 2. Drizzle mushrooms with coconut oil and sprinkle with salt. Scoop ¼ zucchini mixture into each mushroom. 3. Place mushrooms into ungreased air fryer basket. Adjust the temperature to 400°F (204°C) and air fry for 8 minutes. Portobellos will be tender and tops will be browned when done. Serve warm.

Per Serving:

calories: 151 | fat: 13g | protein: 4g | carbs: 6g | fiber: 2g | sodium: 427mg

Chickpea-Spinach Curry

Prep time: 5 minutes | Cook time: 10 minutes |

Serves 2

1 cup frozen chopped spinach, thawed	chopped tomatoes, undrained
1 cup canned chickpeas, drained and rinsed	1 tablespoon curry powder
	1 tablespoon granulated garlic
½ cup frozen green beans	Salt, to season
½ cup frozen broccoli florets	Freshly ground black pepper, to season
½ cup no-salt-added canned	½ cup chopped fresh parsley

1. In a medium saucepan set over high heat, stir together the spinach, chickpeas, green beans, broccoli, tomatoes and their juice, curry powder, and garlic. Season with salt and pepper. Bring to a fast boil. Reduce the heat to low. Cover and simmer for 10 minutes, or until heated through. 2. Top with the parsley, serve, and enjoy!

Per Serving:

calories: 203 | fat: 3g | protein: 13g | carbs: 35g | sugars: 7g | fiber: 13g | sodium: 375mg

The Ultimate Veggie Burger

Prep time: 5 minutes | Cook time: 10 minutes |

Serves 2

¾ cup shelled edamame
¾ cup frozen mixed vegetables, thawed
3 tablespoons hemp hearts
2 tablespoons quick-cook oatmeal
¼ teaspoon salt
¼ teaspoon onion powder

¼ teaspoon ground cumin
1 scallion, sliced
2 teaspoons chopped fresh cilantro
2 tablespoons coconut flour
2 large egg whites
Extra-virgin olive oil cooking spray

1. In a food processor, combine the edamame, mixed vegetables, hemp hearts, oatmeal, salt, onion powder, cumin, scallion, cilantro, coconut flour, and egg whites. Pulse until blended, but not completely puréed. You want some texture. 2. Spray a nonstick skillet with cooking spray. Place it over medium-high heat. 3. Spoon half of the mixture into the pan. Using the back of a spoon, spread it out to form a patty. Repeat with the remaining half of the mixture. 4. Cook for 3 to 5 minutes, or until golden, and flip. Cook for about 3 minutes more, or until golden. Turn off the heat. 5. Transfer to serving plates and enjoy!

Per Serving:

calories: 154 | fat: 4g | protein: 13g | carbs: 19g | sugars: 4g | fiber: 7g | sodium: 467mg

Farro Bowl

Prep time: 5 minutes | Cook time: 25 minutes |

Serves 4

3 cups water
1 cup uncooked farro
1 tablespoon extra-virgin olive oil
1 teaspoon ground cumin
½ teaspoon salt
½ teaspoon freshly ground

black pepper
4 hardboiled eggs, sliced
1 avocado, sliced
⅓ cup plain low-fat Greek yogurt
4 lemon wedges

1. In a medium saucepan, bring the water to a boil over high heat. 2. Pour the farro into the boiling water, and stir to submerge the grains. Reduce the heat to medium and cook for 20 minutes. Drain and set aside. 3. Heat a medium skillet over medium-low heat. When hot, pour in the oil, then add the cooked farro, cumin, salt, and pepper. Cook for 3 to 5 minutes, stirring occasionally. 4. Divide the farro into four equal portions, and top each with one-quarter of the eggs, avocado, and yogurt. Add a squeeze of lemon over the top of each portion.

Per Serving:

calories: 330 | fat: 15g | protein: 14g | carbs: 40g | sugars: 6g | fiber: 8g | sodium: 409mg

Instant Pot Hoppin' John with Skillet Cauli "Rice"

Prep time: 0 minutes | Cook time: 30 minutes |

Serves 6

Hoppin' John
1 pound dried black-eyed peas (about 2¼ cups)
8⅔ cups water
1½ teaspoons fine sea salt
2 tablespoons extra-virgin olive oil
2 garlic cloves, minced
8 ounces shiitake mushrooms, stemmed and chopped, or cremini mushrooms, chopped
1 small yellow onion, diced
1 green bell pepper, seeded and diced
2 celery stalks, diced
2 jalapeño chiles, seeded and

diced
½ teaspoon smoked paprika
½ teaspoon dried thyme
½ teaspoon dried sage
¼ teaspoon cayenne pepper
2 cups low-sodium vegetable broth
Cauli "Rice"
1 tablespoon vegan buttery spread or unsalted butter
1 pound riced cauliflower
½ teaspoon fine sea salt
2 green onions, white and green parts, sliced
Hot sauce (such as Tabasco or Crystal) for serving

1. To make the Hoppin' John: In a large bowl, combine the black-eyed peas, 8 cups of the water, and 1 teaspoon of the salt and stir to dissolve the salt. Let soak for at least 8 hours or up to overnight. 2. Select the Sauté setting on the Instant Pot and heat the oil and garlic for 3 minutes, until the garlic is bubbling but not browned. Add the mushrooms and the remaining ½ teaspoon salt and sauté for 5 minutes, until the mushrooms have wilted and begun to give up their liquid. Add the onion, bell pepper, celery, and jalapeños and sauté for 4 minutes, until the onion is softened. Add the paprika, thyme, sage, and cayenne and sauté for 1 minute. 3. Drain the black-eyed peas and add them to the pot along with the broth and remaining ⅔ cup water. The liquid should just barely cover the beans. (Add an additional splash of water if needed.) 4. Secure the lid and set the Pressure Release to Sealing. Press the Cancel button to reset the cooking program, then select the Bean/Chili, Pressure Cook, or Manual setting and set the cooking time for 5 minutes at high pressure. (The pot will take about 10 minutes to come up to pressure before the cooking program begins.) 5. When the cooking program ends, let the pressure release naturally for 10 minutes, then move the Pressure Release to Venting to release any remaining steam. 6. To make the cauli "rice": While the pressure is releasing, in a large skillet over medium heat, melt the buttery spread. Add the cauliflower and salt and sauté for 3 to 5 minutes, until cooked through and piping hot. (If using frozen riced cauliflower, this may take another 2 minutes or so.) 7. Spoon the cauli "rice" onto individual plates. Open the pot and spoon the black-eyed peas on top of the cauli "rice". Sprinkle with the green onions and serve right away, with the hot sauce on the side.

Per Serving:

calories: 287 | fat: 7g | protein: 23g | carbs: 56g | sugars: 8g | fiber: 24g | sodium: 894mg

Soybeans with Plums and Peppers

Prep time: 15 minutes | Cook time: 40 minutes |
Serves 2

2 medium purple plums
1 tablespoon extra-virgin olive oil
1 medium onion, chopped
1 small yellow bell pepper, chopped
1 small red bell pepper, chopped
1 garlic clove, chopped

2 whole cloves
2 teaspoons ground cumin
½ cup minced fresh cilantro leaves
2 teaspoons freshly squeezed lemon juice
½ teaspoon liquid stevia
1 cup cooked black soybeans

1. Fill a deep pot with water and bring to a boil over high heat. 2. Add the plums. Boil for 30 seconds to loosen their skins. With a slotted spoon, remove the plums. Set aside to cool. 3. In a large skillet set over low heat, heat the olive oil. 4. Add the onion, yellow bell pepper, red bell pepper, garlic, whole cloves, cumin, and cilantro. Cook for 5 to 10 minutes, stirring frequently, until the onion softens. 5. Peel the plums. Remove the pits and chop the fruit. 6. Add the plum, lemon juice, and stevia to the onions and peppers. 7. Stir in the black soybeans. Cover and cook for about 30 minutes, or until the peppers are soft, stirring frequently to prevent sticking. 8. Remove the 2 whole cloves. Serve hot or chilled and enjoy!

Per Serving:

calories: 255 | fat: 5g | protein: 10g | carbs: 46g | sugars: 14g | fiber: 11g | sodium: 22mg

Palak Tofu

Prep time: 5 minutes | Cook time: 40 minutes |
Serves 4

One 14 ounces package extra-firm tofu, drained
5 tablespoons cold-pressed avocado oil
1 yellow onion, diced
1-inch piece fresh ginger, peeled and minced
3 garlic cloves, minced
1 teaspoon fine sea salt
½ teaspoon freshly ground black pepper

¼ teaspoon cayenne pepper
One 16 ounces bag frozen chopped spinach
⅓ cup water
One 14½-ounce can fire-roasted diced tomatoes and their liquid
¼ cup coconut milk
2 teaspoons garam masala
Cooked brown rice or cauliflower "rice" or whole-grain flatbread for serving

1. Cut the tofu crosswise into eight ½-inch-thick slices. Sandwich the slices between double layers of paper towels or a folded kitchen towel and press firmly to wick away as much moisture as possible. Cut the slices into ½-inch cubes. 2. Select the Sauté setting on the Instant Pot and and heat 4 tablespoons of the oil for 2 minutes. Add the onion and sauté for about 10 minutes, until it begins to brown. 3. While the onion is cooking in the Instant Pot, in a large nonstick skillet over medium-high heat, warm the remaining 1 tablespoon oil. Add the tofu in a single layer and cook without stirring for about 3 minutes, until lightly browned. 4. Using a spatula, turn the cubes over and cook for about 3 minutes more, until browned on the other side. Remove from the heat and set aside. 5. Add the ginger and garlic to the onion in the Instant Pot and sauté for about 2 minutes, until the garlic is bubbling but not browned. Add the sautéed tofu, salt, black pepper, and cayenne and stir gently to combine, taking care not to break up the tofu. Add the spinach and stir gently. Pour in the water and then pour the tomatoes and their liquid over the top in an even layer. Do not stir them in. 6. Secure the lid and set the Pressure Release to Sealing. Press the Cancel button to reset the cooking program, then select the Manual or Pressure Cook setting and set the cooking time for 10 minutes at low pressure. (The pot will take about 15 minutes to come up to pressure before the cooking program begins.) 7. When the cooking program ends, let the pressure release naturally for 10 minutes, then move the Pressure Release to Venting to release any remaining steam. Open the pot, add the coconut milk and garam masala, and stir to combine. 8. Ladle the tofu onto plates or into bowls. Serve piping hot, with the "rice" alongside.

Per Serving:

calories: 345 | fat: 24g | protein: 14g | carbs: 18g | sugars: 5g | fiber: 6g | sodium: 777mg

Chickpea and Tofu Bolognese

Prep time: 5 minutes | Cook time: 25 minutes |
Serves 4

1 (3 to 4-pound) spaghetti squash
½ teaspoon ground cumin
1 cup no-sugar-added spaghetti

sauce
1 (15 ounces) can low-sodium chickpeas, drained and rinsed
6 ounces extra-firm tofu

1. Preheat the oven to 400°F. 2. Cut the squash in half lengthwise. Scoop out the seeds and discard. 3. Season both halves of the squash with the cumin, and place them on a baking sheet cut-side down. Roast for 25 minutes. 4. Meanwhile, heat a medium saucepan over low heat, and pour in the spaghetti sauce and chickpeas. 5. Press the tofu between two layers of paper towels, and gently squeeze out any excess water. 6. Crumble the tofu into the sauce and cook for 15 minutes. 7. Remove the squash from the oven, and comb through the flesh of each half with a fork to make thin strands. 8. Divide the "spaghetti" into four portions, and top each portion with one-quarter of the sauce.

Per Serving:

calories: 221 | fat: 6g | protein: 12g | carbs: 32g | sugars: 6g | fiber: 8g | sodium: 405mg

Caprese Eggplant Stacks

Prep time: 5 minutes | Cook time: 12 minutes | Serves 4

1 medium eggplant, cut into ¼-inch slices
2 large tomatoes, cut into ¼-inch slices
4 ounces (113 g) fresh Mozzarella, cut into ½-ounce / 14-g slices

2 tablespoons olive oil
¼ cup fresh basil, sliced

1. In a baking dish, place four slices of eggplant on the bottom. Place a slice of tomato on top of each eggplant round, then Mozzarella, then eggplant. Repeat as necessary. 2. Drizzle with olive oil. Cover dish with foil and place dish into the air fryer basket. 3. Adjust the temperature to 350ºF (177ºC) and bake for 12 minutes. 4. When done, eggplant will be tender. Garnish with fresh basil to serve.

Per Serving:

calories: 97 | fat: 7g | protein: 2g | carbs: 8g | fiber: 4g | sodium: 11mg

Southwest Tofu

Prep time: 10 minutes | Cook time: 20 minutes | Serves 4

3½ tablespoons freshly squeezed lime juice
2 teaspoons pure maple syrup
1½ teaspoons ground cumin
1 teaspoon dried oregano leaves
1 teaspoon chili powder
½ teaspoon paprika

½ teaspoon sea salt
⅛ teaspoon allspice
1 package (12 ounces) extra-firm tofu, sliced into ¼"–½" thick squares and patted to remove excess moisture

1. In a 9" x 12" baking dish, combine the lime juice, syrup, cumin, oregano, chili powder, paprika, salt, and allspice. Add the tofu and turn to coat both sides. Bake uncovered for 20 minutes, or until the marinade is absorbed, turning once.

Per Serving:

calorie: 78 | fat: 4g | protein: 7g | carbs: 6g | sugars: 3g | fiber: 1g | sodium: 324mg

Chapter 10 Stews and Soups

Comforting Chicken and Mushroom Soup

Prep time: 5 minutes | Cook time: 20 minutes |

Serves 6

1 quart low-sodium chicken broth	1 tablespoon finely chopped scallions
1 tablespoon light soy sauce	1 tablespoon dry sherry
1 cup sliced mushrooms, stems removed	½ pound boneless, skinless chicken breast, cubed

1. In a stockpot, simmer all ingredients except the chicken for 10 minutes. 2. Add the chicken cubes, and simmer for 6 to 8 minutes more. Serve with additional soy sauce if desired (but be aware that this will raise the sodium level of the soup).

Per Serving:

calories: 88 | fat: 4g | protein: 10g | carbs: 2g | sugars: 1g | fiber: 0g | sodium: 88mg

Savory Beef Stew with Mushrooms and Turnips

Prep time: 0 minutes | Cook time: 55 minutes |

Serves 6

1½ pounds beef stew meat	sauce
¾ teaspoon fine sea salt	1 tablespoon Dijon mustard
¾ teaspoon freshly ground black pepper	1 teaspoon dried rosemary, crumbled
1 tablespoon cold-pressed avocado oil	1 bay leaf
3 garlic cloves, minced	3 tablespoons tomato paste
1 yellow onion, diced	8 ounces carrots, cut into 1-inch-thick rounds
2 celery stalks, diced	1 pound turnips, cut into 1-inch pieces
8 ounces cremini mushrooms, quartered	1 pound parsnips, halved lengthwise, then cut crosswise into 1-inch pieces
1 cup low-sodium roasted beef bone broth	
2 tablespoons Worcestershire	

1. Sprinkle the beef all over with the salt and pepper. 2. Select the Sauté setting on the Instant Pot and heat the oil and garlic for 2 minutes, until the garlic is bubbling but not browned. Add the onion, celery, and mushrooms and sauté for 5 minutes, until the onion begins to soften and the mushrooms are giving up their liquid. Stir in the broth, Worcestershire sauce, mustard, rosemary, and bay leaf. Stir in the beef. Add the tomato paste in a dollop on top. Do not stir it in. 3. Secure the lid and set the Pressure Release to Sealing. Press the Cancel button to reset the cooking program, then select the Meat/Stew, Pressure Cook, or Manual setting and set the cooking time for 20 minutes at high pressure. (The pot will take about 10 minutes to come up to pressure before the cooking program begins.) 4. When the cooking program ends, perform a quick pressure release by moving the Pressure Release to Venting, or let the pressure release naturally. Open the pot, remove and discard the bay leaf, and stir in the tomato paste. Place the carrots, turnips, and parsnips on top of the meat. 5. Secure the lid and set the Pressure Release to Sealing. Press the Cancel button to reset the cooking program, then select the Pressure Cook or Manual setting and set the cooking time for 3 minutes at low pressure. (The pot will take about 15 minutes to come up to pressure before the cooking program begins.) 6. When the cooking program ends, perform a quick pressure release by moving the Pressure Release to Venting. Open the pot and stir to combine all of the ingredients. 7. Ladle the stew into bowls and serve hot.

Per Serving:

calories: 304 | fat: 8g | protein: 29g | carbs: 30g | sugars: 10g | fiber: 8g | sodium: 490mg

Gazpacho

Prep time: 15 minutes | Cook time: 0 minutes |

Serves 4

3 pounds ripe tomatoes, chopped	parsley
1 cup low-sodium tomato juice	2 garlic cloves, chopped
½ red onion, chopped	2 tablespoons extra-virgin olive oil
1 cucumber, peeled, seeded, and chopped	2 tablespoons red wine vinegar
1 red bell pepper, seeded and chopped	1 teaspoon honey
2 celery stalks, chopped	½ teaspoon salt
2 tablespoons chopped fresh	¼ teaspoon freshly ground black pepper

1. In a blender jar, combine the tomatoes, tomato juice, onion, cucumber, bell pepper, celery, parsley, garlic, olive oil, vinegar, honey, salt, and pepper. Pulse until blended but still slightly chunky. 2. Adjust the seasonings as needed and serve. 3. To store, transfer to a nonreactive, airtight container and refrigerate for up to 3 days.

Per Serving:

calories: 170 | fat: 8g | protein: 5g | carbs: 24g | sugars: 16g | fiber: 6g | sodium: 332mg

Cauli-Curry Bean Soup

Prep time: 10 minutes | Cook time: 25 minutes | Serves 8

2 cups chopped onion
1½ cups chopped carrot or sweet potato
1½ tablespoons curry powder (or to taste; use more if you really love curry)
1¼ teaspoons sea salt
Freshly ground black pepper to taste
1 teaspoon mustard seeds
1 teaspoon ground cumin
1 teaspoon ground turmeric
¼ teaspoon ground cardamom
⅛ teaspoon ground cinnamon

4 to 5 tablespoons + 4 cups water
3 to 4 cups cauliflower florets
1 can (15 ounces) chickpeas, rinsed and drained
1 can (15 ounces) adzuki or black beans, rinsed and drained
1 cup dried red lentils
1 can (28 ounces) crushed tomatoes
1 tablespoon grated fresh ginger
1 to 2 teaspoons pure maple syrup (optional)

1. In a large pot over medium-high heat, combine the onion, carrot or sweet potato, curry powder, salt, pepper, mustard seeds, cumin, turmeric, cardamom, cinnamon, and 3 tablespoons of the water. Stir, cover, and cook for 4 to 5 minutes, stirring occasionally. (Add another 1 to 2 tablespoons of water if needed to keep the vegetables and spices from sticking.) Add the cauliflower, chickpeas, beans, lentils, tomatoes, and remaining 4 cups water. Stir and increase the heat to high to bring to a boil. Reduce the heat to low, cover, and simmer for 15 to 20 minutes. Stir in the ginger and syrup (if using). Season to taste, and serve.

Per Serving:

calorie: 226 | fat: 2g | protein: 14g | carbs: 42g | sugars: 7g | fiber: 13g | sodium: 577mg

French Market Soup

Prep time: 20 minutes | Cook time: 1 hour | Serves 8

2 cups mixed dry beans, washed with stones removed
7 cups water
1 ham hock, all visible fat removed
1 teaspoon salt
¼ teaspoon pepper

16 ounces can low-sodium tomatoes
1 large onion, chopped
1 garlic clove, minced
1 chile, chopped, or 1 teaspoon chili powder
¼ cup lemon juice

1. Combine all ingredients in the inner pot of the Instant Pot. 2. Secure the lid and make sure vent is set to sealing. Using Manual, set the Instant Pot to cook for 60 minutes. 3. When cooking time is over, let the pressure release naturally. When the Instant Pot is ready, unlock the lid, then remove the bone and any hard or fatty pieces. Pull the meat off the bone and chop into small pieces. Add the ham back into the Instant Pot.

Per Serving:

calories: 191 | fat: 4g | protein: 12g | carbs: 29g | sugars: 5g | fiber: 7g | sodium: 488mg

Chock-Full-of-Vegetables Chicken Soup

Prep time: 5 minutes | Cook time: 15 minutes | Serves 2

1 tablespoon extra-virgin olive oil
8 ounces chicken tenders, cut into bite-size chunks
1 small zucchini, finely diced
1 cup sliced fresh button mushrooms
2 medium carrots, thinly sliced
2 celery stalks, thinly sliced

1 large shallot, finely chopped
1 garlic clove, minced
1 tablespoon dried parsley
1 teaspoon dried marjoram
⅛ teaspoon salt
2 plum tomatoes, chopped
2 cups reduced-sodium chicken broth
1½ cups packed baby spinach

1. In a large saucepan set over medium-high heat, heat olive oil. 2. Add the chicken. Cook for 3 to 4 minutes, stirring occasionally, or until browned. Transfer to a plate. Set aside. 3. To the saucepan, add the zucchini, mushrooms, carrots, celery, shallot, garlic, parsley, marjoram, and salt. Cook for 2 to 3 minutes, stirring frequently, until the vegetables are slightly softened. 4. Add the tomatoes and chicken broth. Increase the heat to high. Bring to a boil, stirring occasionally. Reduce the heat to low. Simmer for 5 minutes, or until the vegetables are tender. 5. Stir in the spinach, cooked chicken, and any accumulated juices on the plate. Cook for about 2 minutes, stirring, until the chicken is heated through. 6. Serve hot and enjoy!

Per Serving:

calories: 262 | fat: 9.56g | protein: 31.94g | carbs: 15.57g | sugars: 2.58g | fiber: 6.2g | sodium: 890mg

White Bean Soup

Prep time: 15 minutes | Cook time: 20 minutes | Serves 2

1 teaspoon extra-virgin olive oil
⅓ cup chopped yellow onion
1 garlic clove, minced
1 teaspoon dried rosemary
½ cup sliced fresh mushrooms
½ cup jarred roasted red peppers, chopped
1 teaspoon freshly squeezed

lemon juice
1 teaspoon white wine vinegar
1 cup water
1 (15 ounces) can white beans, drained and rinsed
½ cup diced tomatoes, with juice
1½ cups fresh spinach

1. In a large pot set over medium heat, heat the olive oil. 2. Add the onion and garlic. Sauté for about 5 minutes, or until tender. 3. Add the rosemary, mushrooms, red peppers, lemon juice, white wine vinegar, and water. Cook for 5 minutes more, or until the mushrooms are soft. 4. Stir in the white beans, tomatoes, and spinach. Cook for 10 minutes more, or until the spinach is wilted. 5. Serve immediately and enjoy!

Per Serving:

calories: 96 | fat: 4.73g | protein: 3.19g | carbs: 12.65g | sugars: 4.41g | fiber: 4.4g | sodium: 28mg

Cauliflower Chili

Prep time: 10 minutes | Cook time: 35 minutes |
Serves 5

2 cups thickly sliced carrot
½ large or 1 full small head cauliflower
4 or 5 cloves garlic, minced
1 tablespoon balsamic vinegar
1½ cups diced onion
1 teaspoon sea salt
1½ tablespoons mild chili powder
1 tablespoon cocoa powder
2 teaspoons ground cumin
2 teaspoons dried oregano

⅛ teaspoon allspice
¼ teaspoon crushed red-pepper flakes (or to taste)
1 can (28 ounces) crushed tomatoes
1 can (15 ounces) pinto beans, rinsed and drained
1 can (15 ounces) kidney beans or black beans, rinsed and drained
½ cup water
Lime wedges

1. In a food processor, combine the carrot, cauliflower, and garlic, and pulse until finely minced. (Alternatively, you could mince by hand.) In a large pot over medium heat, combine the vinegar, onion, salt, chili powder, cocoa, cumin, oregano, allspice, and red-pepper flakes. Cook for 3 to 4 minutes, stirring occasionally. Add the minced carrot, cauliflower, and garlic, and cook for 5 to 6 minutes, stirring occasionally. Add the tomatoes, pinto and kidney beans, and water, and stir to combine. Increase the heat to high to bring to a boil. Reduce the heat to low, cover, and simmer for 25 minutes. Taste, and season as desired. Serve with lime wedges.

Per Serving:

calorie: 237 | fat: 3g | protein: 13g | carbs: 45g | sugars: 13g | fiber: 15g | sodium: 1036mg

Asparagus Soup

Prep time: 5 minutes | Cook time: 10 minutes |
Serves 2

1 pound asparagus, woody ends removed, sliced into 1-inch pieces
1 (8 ounces) can cannellini beans, drained and rinsed
2 cups reduced-sodium vegetable broth
1 medium shallot, thinly sliced

1 garlic clove, thinly sliced
½ teaspoon dried thyme
½ teaspoon dried marjoram leaves
⅛ teaspoon salt
Freshly ground black pepper, to season

1. In a large saucepan set over high heat, stir together the asparagus, cannellini beans, vegetable broth, shallot, garlic, thyme, marjoram, and salt. Bring to a boil. Reduce the heat to medium-low. Cover and simmer for about 5 minutes, or until the asparagus is tender. 2. In a large blender or food processor, purée the soup until smooth, scraping down the sides, if necessary. Season with pepper. 3. Serve immediately and enjoy!

Per Serving:

calories: 83 | fat: 1g | protein: 6g | carbs: 17g | sugars: 7g | fiber: 7g | sodium: 712mg

Tasty Tomato Soup

Prep time: 10 minutes | Cook time: 1 hour 25
minutes | Serves 2

3 cups chopped tomatoes
1 red bell pepper, cut into chunks
2 tablespoons extra-virgin olive oil, divided
Salt, to season
Freshly ground black pepper, to season

1 medium onion, chopped
1 garlic clove, minced
2 cups low-sodium vegetable broth
1 cup sliced fresh button mushrooms
½ cup fresh chopped basil

1. Preheat the oven to 400°F. 2. On a baking sheet, spread out the tomatoes and red bell pepper. 3. Drizzle with 1 tablespoon of olive oil. Toss to coat. Season with salt and pepper. Place the sheet in the preheated oven. Roast for 45 minutes. 4. In a large stockpot set over medium heat, heat the remaining 1 tablespoon of olive oil. 5. Add the onion. Cook for 2 to 3 minutes, or until tender. 6. Stir in the garlic. Cook for 2 minutes more. 7. Add the vegetable broth, mushrooms, and basil. 8. Stir in the roasted tomatoes and peppers. Reduce the heat to medium-low. Cook for 30 minutes. 9. To a blender or food processor, carefully transfer the soup in batches, blending until smooth. Return the processed soup to the pot. Simmer for 5 minutes. 10. Serve warm and enjoy!

Per Serving:

calories: 255 | fat: 15g | protein: 6g | carbs: 29g | sugars: 18g | fiber: 7g | sodium: 738mg

Herbed Chicken Stew with Noodles

Prep time: 10 minutes | Cook time: 40 minutes |
Serves 8

1 tablespoon extra-virgin olive oil
1 onion, chopped
2 garlic cloves, minced
1 pound boneless, skinless chicken breast, cubed
2 tablespoons flour
3 cups low-sodium chicken

broth
1 cup dry white wine
1 tablespoon chopped fresh thyme (or 1 teaspoon dried)
4 cups cooked egg noodles, hot (from 1/2 pound dry egg noodles)
½ cup minced parsley

1. In a large saucepan, heat the oil and sauté the onion and garlic for about 5 minutes. Add the chicken cubes, and sauté until the chicken is cooked (about 10 minutes). 2. Sprinkle the flour over the chicken. Add the chicken broth, wine, and thyme. Bring to a boil, and then lower the heat and simmer for 30 minutes. 3. Toss together the noodles and the parsley in a large bowl. Pour the stew over the noodles and serve.

Per Serving:

calories: 285 | fat: 9g | protein: 14g | carbs: 37g | sugars: 4g | fiber: 2g | sodium: 419mg

Beef, Mushroom, and Wild Rice Soup

Prep time: 0 minutes | Cook time: 55 minutes |

Serves 6

2 tablespoons extra-virgin olive oil or unsalted butter	1½ pounds beef stew meat, larger pieces halved, or beef chuck, trimmed of fat and cut into ¾-inch pieces
2 garlic cloves, minced	
8 ounces shiitake mushrooms, stems removed and sliced	
1 teaspoon fine sea salt	4 cups low-sodium roasted beef bone broth
2 carrots, diced	1 cup wild rice, rinsed
2 celery stalks, diced	1 tablespoon Worcestershire sauce
1 yellow onion, diced	
1 teaspoon dried thyme	2 tablespoons tomato paste

1. Select the Sauté setting on the Instant Pot and heat the oil and garlic for about 1 minute, until the garlic is bubbling but not browned. Add the mushrooms and salt and sauté for 5 minutes, until the mushrooms have wilted and given up some of their liquid. Add the carrots, celery, and onion and sauté for 4 minutes, until the onion begins to soften. Add the thyme and beef and sauté for 3 minutes more, until the beef is mostly opaque on the outside. Stir in the broth, rice, Worcestershire sauce, and tomato paste, using a wooden spoon to nudge any browned bits from the bottom of the pot. 2. Secure the lid and set the Pressure Release to Sealing. Press the Cancel button to reset the cooking program, then select the Pressure Cook or Manual setting and set the cooking time for 25 minutes at high pressure. (The pot will take about 15 minutes to come up to pressure before the cooking program begins.) 3. When the cooking program ends, let the pressure release naturally for at least 15 minutes, then move the Pressure Release to Venting to release any remaining steam. Open the pot. Ladle the soup into bowls and serve hot.

Per Serving:

calories: 316 | fat: 8g | protein: 29g | carbs: 32g | sugars: 6g | fiber: 8g | sodium: 783mg

Hearty Hamburger and Lentil Stew

Prep time: 0 minutes | Cook time: 55 minutes |

Serves 8

2 tablespoons cold-pressed avocado oil	1 tablespoon Italian seasoning
2 garlic cloves, chopped	1 tablespoon paprika
1 large yellow onion, diced	1½ teaspoons fine sea salt
2 carrots, diced	1 extra-large russet potato, diced
2 celery stalks, diced	
2 pounds 95 percent lean ground beef	1 cup frozen green peas
	1 cup frozen corn
½ cup small green lentils	One 14½-ounce can no-salt petite diced tomatoes and their liquid
2 cups low-sodium roasted beef bone broth or vegetable broth	
	¼ cup tomato paste

1. Select the Sauté setting on the Instant Pot and heat the oil and garlic for 3 minutes, until the garlic is bubbling but not browned. Add the onion, carrots, and celery and sauté for 5 minutes, until the onion begins to soften. Add the beef and sauté, using a wooden spoon or spatula to break up the meat as it cooks, for 6 minutes, until cooked through and no streaks of pink remain. 2. Stir in the lentils, broth, Italian seasoning, paprika, and salt. Add the potato, peas, corn, and tomatoes and their liquid in layers on top of the lentils and beef, then add the tomato paste in a dollop on top. Do not stir in the vegetables and tomato paste. 3. Secure the lid and set the Pressure Release to Sealing. Press the Cancel button to reset the cooking program, then select the Pressure Cook or Manual setting and set the cooking time for 20 minutes at high pressure. (The pot will take about 20 minutes to come up to pressure before the cooking program begins.) 4. When the cooking program ends, let the pressure release naturally for at least 15 minutes, then move the Pressure Release to Venting to release any remaining steam. Open the pot and stir the stew to mix all of the ingredients. 5. Ladle the stew into bowls and serve hot.

Per Serving:

calories: 334 | fat: 8g | protein: 34g | carbs: 30g | sugars: 6g | fiber: 7g | sodium: 902mg

Chicken Brunswick Stew

Prep time: 0 minutes | Cook time: 30 minutes |

Serves 6

2 tablespoons extra-virgin olive oil	1 cup low-sodium chicken broth
2 garlic cloves, chopped	1 tablespoon hot sauce (such as Tabasco or Crystal)
1 large yellow onion, diced	
2 pounds boneless, skinless chicken (breasts, tenders, or thighs), cut into bite-size pieces	1 tablespoon raw apple cider vinegar
	1½ cups frozen corn
1 teaspoon dried thyme	1½ cups frozen baby lima beans
1 teaspoon smoked paprika	One 14½-ounce can fire-roasted diced tomatoes and their liquid
1 teaspoon fine sea salt	
½ teaspoon freshly ground black pepper	2 tablespoons tomato paste
	Cornbread, for serving

1. Select the Sauté setting on the Instant Pot and heat the oil and garlic for 2 minutes, until the garlic is bubbling but not browned. Add the onion and sauté for 3 minutes, until it begins to soften. Add the chicken and sauté for 3 minutes more, until mostly opaque. The chicken does not have to be cooked through. Add the thyme, paprika, salt, and pepper and sauté for 1 minute more. 2. Stir in the broth, hot sauce, vinegar, corn, and lima beans. Add the diced tomatoes and their liquid in an even layer and dollop the tomato paste on top. Do not stir them in. 3. Secure the lid and set the Pressure Release to Sealing. Press the Cancel button to reset the cooking program, then select the Pressure Cook or Manual setting and set the cooking time for 5 minutes at high pressure. (The pot will take about 15 minutes to come up to pressure before the cooking program begins.) 4. When the cooking program ends, let the pressure release naturally for at least 10 minutes, then move the Pressure Release to Venting to release any remaining steam. Open the pot and stir the stew to mix all of the ingredients. 5. Ladle the stew into bowls and serve hot, with cornbread alongside.

Per Serving:

calories: 349 | fat: 7g | protein: 40g | carbs: 17g | sugars: 7g | fiber: 7g | sodium: 535mg

Unstuffed Cabbage Soup

Prep time: 15 minutes | Cook time: 20 minutes |

Serves 5

2 tablespoons coconut oil
1 pound ground sirloin or turkey
1 medium onion, diced
2 cloves garlic, minced
1 small head cabbage, chopped, cored, cut into roughly 2-inch pieces.
6 ounces can low-sodium tomato paste

32 ounces can low-sodium diced tomatoes, with liquid
2 cups low-sodium beef broth
1½ cups water
¾ cup brown rice
1 to 2 teaspoons salt
½ teaspoon black pepper
1 teaspoon oregano
1 teaspoon parsley

1. Melt coconut oil in the inner pot of the Instant Pot using Sauté function. Add ground meat. Stir frequently until meat loses color, about 2 minutes. 2. Add onion and garlic and continue to sauté for 2 more minutes, stirring frequently. 3. Add chopped cabbage. 4. On top of cabbage layer tomato paste, tomatoes with liquid, beef broth, water, rice, and spices. 5. Secure the lid and set vent to sealing. Using Manual setting, select 20 minutes. 6. When time is up, let the pressure release naturally for 10 minutes, then do a quick release.

Per Serving:

calories: 282 | fat: 6g | protein: 23g | carbs: 34g | sugars: 6g | fiber: 3g | sodium: 898mg

Lentil Stew

Prep time: 10 minutes | Cook time: 30 minutes |

Serves 2

½ cup dry lentils, picked through, debris removed, rinsed and drained
2½ cups water
1 bay leaf
2 teaspoons dried tarragon
2 teaspoons dried thyme
2 garlic cloves, minced
2 medium carrots, chopped

2 medium tomatoes, diced
1 celery stalk, chopped
1 tablespoon extra-virgin olive oil
1 medium onion, diced
1 cup frozen spinach
Salt, to season
Freshly ground black pepper, to season

1. In a soup pot set over high heat, stir together the lentils, water, bay leaf, tarragon, thyme, and garlic. 2. Add the carrots, tomatoes, and celery. Cover. Bring to a boil. Reduce the heat to low and stir the soup. Simmer for 15 to 20 minutes, covered, or until the lentils are tender. 3. While the vegetables simmer, place a skillet over medium heat. Add the olive oil and onion. Sauté for about 10 minutes, or until browned. Remove the skillet from the heat. 4. When the lentils are tender, remove and discard the bay leaf. Add the cooked onion and the spinach to the soup. Heat for 5 to 10 minutes more, or until the spinach is cooked. 5. Season with salt and pepper. 6. Enjoy immediately.

Per Serving:

calories: 214 | fat: 7g | protein: 10g | carbs: 31g | sugars: 10g | fiber: 11g | sodium: 871mg

Green Chile Corn Chowder

Prep time: 20 minutes | Cook time: 7 to 8 hours |

Serves 8

16 ounces can cream-style corn
3 potatoes, peeled and diced
2 tablespoons chopped fresh chives
4 ounces can diced green chilies, drained
2 ounces jar chopped pimentos, drained

½ cup chopped cooked ham
Two 10½ ounces cans 100% fat-free lower-sodium chicken broth
Pepper to taste
Tabasco sauce to taste
1 cup fat-free milk

1. Combine all ingredients, except milk, in the inner pot of the Instant Pot. 2. Secure the lid and cook using the Slow Cook function on low 7 to 8 hours or until potatoes are tender. 3. When cook time is up, remove the lid and stir in the milk. Cover and let simmer another 20 minutes.

Per Serving:

calories: 124 | fat: 2g | protein: 6g | carbs: 21g | sugars: 7g | fiber: 2g | sodium: 563mg

Chicken Tortilla Soup

Prep time: 10 minutes | Cook time: 35 minutes |

Serves 4

1 tablespoon extra-virgin olive oil
1 onion, thinly sliced
1 garlic clove, minced
1 jalapeño pepper, diced
2 boneless, skinless chicken breasts
4 cups low-sodium chicken broth
1 roma tomato, diced

½ teaspoon salt
2 (6-inch) corn tortillas, cut into thin strips
Nonstick cooking spray
Juice of 1 lime
Minced fresh cilantro, for garnish
¼ cup shredded cheddar cheese, for garnish

1. In a medium pot, heat the oil over medium-high heat. Add the onion and cook for 3 to 5 minutes until it begins to soften. Add the garlic and jalapeño, and cook until fragrant, about 1 minute more. 2. Add the chicken, chicken broth, tomato, and salt to the pot and bring to a boil. Reduce the heat to medium and simmer gently for 20 to 25 minutes until the chicken breasts are cooked through. Remove the chicken from the pot and set aside. 3. Preheat a broiler to high. 4. Spray the tortilla strips with nonstick cooking spray and toss to coat. Spread in a single layer on a baking sheet and broil for 3 to 5 minutes, flipping once, until crisp. 5. When the chicken is cool enough to handle, shred it with two forks and return to the pot. 6. Season the soup with the lime juice. Serve hot, garnished with cilantro, cheese, and tortilla strips.

Per Serving:

calories: 191 | fat: 8g | protein: 19g | carbs: 13g | sugars: 2g | fiber: 2g | sodium: 482mg

Italian Vegetable Soup

Prep time: 20 minutes | Cook time: 5 to 9 hours |

Serves 6

3 small carrots, sliced
1 small onion, chopped
2 small potatoes, diced
2 tablespoons chopped parsley
1 garlic clove, minced
3 teaspoons sodium-free beef bouillon powder
1¼ teaspoons dried basil

¼ teaspoon pepper
16 ounces can red kidney beans, undrained
3 cups water
14½-ounce can stewed tomatoes, with juice
1 cup diced, extra-lean, lower-sodium cooked ham

1. In the inner pot of the Instant Pot, layer the carrots, onion, potatoes, parsley, garlic, beef bouillon, basil, pepper, and kidney beans. Do not stir. Add water. 2. Secure the lid and cook on the Low Slow Cook mode for 8 to 9 hours, or on high 4½ to 5½ hours, until vegetables are tender. 3. Remove the lid and stir in the tomatoes and ham. Secure the lid again and cook on high Slow Cook mode for 10–15 minutes more.

Per Serving:

calories: 156 | fat: 1g | protein: 9g | carbs: 29g | sugars: 8g | fiber: 5g | sodium: 614mg

Quick Moroccan-Inspired Chicken Stew

Prep time: 5 minutes | Cook time: 15 minutes |

Serves 4 to 6

2 teaspoons ground cumin
1 teaspoon ground cinnamon
½ teaspoon turmeric
½ teaspoon paprika
1½ pounds boneless, skinless chicken, cut into strips
2 tablespoons extra-virgin olive oil

5 garlic cloves, smashed and coarsely chopped
2 onions, thinly sliced
1 tablespoon fresh lemon zest
½ cup coarsely chopped olives
2 cups low-sodium chicken broth
Cilantro, for garnish (optional)

1. In a medium bowl, mix together the cumin, cinnamon, turmeric, and paprika until well blended. Add the chicken, tossing to coat, and set aside. 2. Heat the extra-virgin olive oil in a large skillet or medium Dutch oven over medium-high heat. Add the chicken and garlic in one layer and cook, browning on all sides, about 2 minutes. 3. Add the onions, lemon zest, olives, and broth and bring the soup to a boil. Reduce the heat to medium low, cover, and simmer for 8 minutes. 4. Uncover the soup and let it simmer for another 2 to 3 minutes for the sauce to thicken slightly. Adjust the seasonings as desired and serve garnished with cilantro (if using). 5. Store the cooled soup in an airtight container in the refrigerator for up to 5 days.

Per Serving:

calories: 252 | fat: 10g | protein: 13g | carbs: 28g | sugars: 6g | fiber: 3g | sodium: 451mg

Potlikker Soup

Prep time: 15 minutes | Cook time: 20 minutes |

Serves 6

3 cups store-bought low-sodium chicken broth, divided
1 medium onion, chopped
3 garlic cloves, minced
1 bunch collard greens or mustard greens including stems, roughly chopped

1 fresh ham bone
5 carrots, peeled and cut into 1-inch rounds
2 fresh thyme sprigs
3 bay leaves
Freshly ground black pepper

1. Select the Sauté setting on an electric pressure cooker, and combine ½ cup of chicken broth, the onion, and garlic and cook for 3 to 5 minutes, or until the onion and garlic are translucent. 2. Add the collard greens, ham bone, carrots, remaining 2½ cups of broth, the thyme, and bay leaves. 3. Close and lock the lid and set the pressure valve to sealing. 4. Change to the Manual/Pressure Cook setting, and cook for 15 minutes. 5. Once cooking is complete, quick-release the pressure. Carefully remove the lid. Discard the bay leaves. 6. Serve.

Per Serving:

calories: 107 | fat: 3g | protein: 12g | carbs: 12g | sugars: 3g | fiber: 5g | sodium: 556mg

Hearty Italian Minestrone

Prep time: 10 minutes | Cook time: 50 minutes |

Serves 8

½ cup sliced onion
1 tablespoon extra-virgin olive oil
4 cups low-sodium chicken broth
¾ cup diced carrot
½ cup diced potato (with skin)
2 cups sliced cabbage or coarsely chopped spinach
1 cup diced zucchini
½ cup cooked garbanzo beans (drained and rinsed, if canned)

½ cup cooked navy beans (drained and rinsed, if canned)
One 14½ ounces can low-sodium tomatoes, with liquid
½ cup diced celery
2 tablespoons fresh basil, finely chopped
½ cup uncooked whole-wheat rotini or other shaped pasta
2 tablespoons fresh parsley, finely chopped, for garnish

1. In a large stockpot over medium heat, sauté the onion in oil until the onion is slightly browned. Add the chicken broth, carrot, and potato. Cover and cook over medium heat for 30 minutes. 2. Add the remaining ingredients and cook for an additional 15–20 minutes, until the pasta is cooked through. Garnish with parsley and serve hot.

Per Serving:

calories: 101 | fat: 2.01g | protein: 5.86g | carbs: 16.51g | sugars: 4.45g | fiber: 3.9g | sodium: 108mg

Instantly Good Beef Stew

Prep time: 20 minutes | Cook time: 35 minutes |
Serves 6

3 tablespoons olive oil,divided
2 pounds stewing beef, cubed
2 cloves garlic, minced
1 large onion, chopped
3 ribs celery, sliced
3 large potatoes, cubed
2 to 3 carrots, sliced
8 ounces no-salt-added tomato

sauce
10 ounces low-sodium beef broth
2 teaspoons Worcestershire sauce
¼ teaspoon pepper
1 bay leaf

1. Set the Instant Pot to the Sauté function, then add in 1 tablespoon of the oil. Add in ⅓ of the beef cubes and brown and sear all sides. Repeat this process twice more with the remaining oil and beef cubes. Set the beef aside. 2. Place the garlic, onion, and celery into the pot and sauté for a few minutes. Press Cancel. 3. Add the beef back in as well as all of the remaining ingredients. 4. Secure the lid and make sure the vent is set to sealing. Choose Manual for 35 minutes. 5. When cook time is up, let the pressure release naturally for 15 minutes, then release any remaining pressure manually. 6. Remove the lid, remove the bay leaf, then serve.

Per Serving:
calories: 401 | fat: 20g | protein: 35g | carbs: 19g | sugars: 5g | fiber: 3g | sodium: 157mg

Freshened-Up French Onion Soup

Prep time: 15 minutes | Cook time: 30 minutes |
Serves 2

1 tablespoon extra-virgin olive oil
2 medium onions, sliced
2 cups low-sodium beef broth
1 (8 ounces) can chickpeas, drained and rinsed

½ teaspoon dried thyme
Salt
Freshly ground black pepper
4 slices nonfat Swiss deli-style cheese

1. In a medium soup pot set over medium-low heat, heat the olive oil. 2. Add the onions. Stir to coat them in oil. Cook for about 10 minutes, or until golden brown. 3. Add the beef broth, chickpeas, and thyme. Bring to a simmer. 4. Taste the broth. Season with salt and pepper. Cook for 10 minutes more. 5. Preheat the broiler to high. 6. Ladle the soup into 2 ovenproof soup bowls. 7. Top each with 2 slices of Swiss cheese. Place the bowls on a baking sheet. Carefully transfer the sheet to the preheated oven. Melt the cheese under the broiler for 2 minutes. Alternately, you can melt the cheese in the microwave (in microwave-safe bowls) on high in 30-second intervals until melted. 8. Enjoy immediately.

Per Serving:
calories: 278 | fat: 14g | protein: 15g | carbs: 29g | sugars: 3g | fiber: 2g | sodium: 804mg

Cheeseburger Soup

Prep time: 5 minutes | Cook time: 25 minutes |
Serves 4

Avocado oil cooking spray
½ cup diced white onion
½ cup diced celery
½ cup sliced portobello mushrooms
1 pound 93% lean ground beef

1 (15 ounces) can no-salt-added diced tomatoes
2 cups low-sodium beef broth
⅓ cup half-and-half
¾ cup shredded sharp Cheddar cheese

1. Heat a large stockpot over medium-low heat. When hot, coat the cooking surface with cooking spray. Put the onion, celery, and mushrooms into the pot. Cook for 7 minutes, stirring occasionally. 2. Add the ground beef and cook for 5 minutes, stirring and breaking apart as needed. 3. Add the diced tomatoes with their juices and the broth. Increase the heat to medium-high and simmer for 10 minutes. 4. Remove the pot from the heat and stir in the half-and-half. 5. Serve topped with the cheese.

Per Serving:
calories: 423 | fat: 21g | protein: 39g | carbs: 22g | sugars: 7g | fiber: 3g | sodium: 171mg

High-Fiber Pumpkin-Cashew Soup

Prep time: 10 minutes | Cook time: 22 minutes |
Serves 4

1 tablespoon (15 ml) olive oil
3 medium carrots, coarsely chopped
1 medium onion, coarsely chopped
1 tablespoon (6 g) grated fresh ginger or ¼ teaspoon ground ginger
1 teaspoon ground cinnamon
½ teaspoon ground cumin
½ teaspoon ground nutmeg

1 (15 ounces [425 g]) can pumpkin purée
2 cups (480 ml) low-sodium vegetable broth
1 cup (240 ml) plain unsweetened almond milk
½ cup (55 g) raw cashews
½ (15 ounces [425 g]) can navy beans, undrained
1 teaspoon apple cider vinegar

1. Heat the oil in a large pot over medium heat. 2. Add the carrots, onion, ginger, cinnamon, cumin, and nutmeg. Sauté this mixture for 5 to 7 minutes, or until the onion is translucent. 3. Add the pumpkin purée, broth, and almond milk and stir to combine. 4. Simmer the soup for 15 minutes, or until the carrots are soft. 5. Let the soup cool slightly, then transfer it to a high-power blender and add the cashews, beans and their liquid, and vinegar. Blend the soup until it is smooth and creamy. Serve the soup immediately, or freeze it in smaller portions for future use.

Per Serving:
calorie: 260 | fat: 12g | protein: 9g | carbs: 34g | sugars: 11g | fiber: 9g | sodium: 152mg

Black Bean Soup with Sweet Potatoes

Prep time: 10 minutes | Cook time: 30 minutes |

Serves 4

1 tablespoon balsamic vinegar	4 medium-large cloves garlic,
1½ to 1¾ cups chopped onion	minced or grated
1½ cups combination of	2 tablespoons tomato paste
chopped red and green bell	2 tablespoons freshly squeezed
peppers	lime juice
1 teaspoon sea salt	½ to 1 teaspoon pure maple
Freshly ground black pepper to	syrup
taste	4½ cups (about 3 cans, 15
2 teaspoons cumin seeds	ounces each) black beans,
2 teaspoons dried oregano	drained and rinsed
leaves	1 bay leaf
Rounded ¼ teaspoon allspice	1½ cups ½" cubes yellow sweet
¼ teaspoon red-pepper flakes,	potato (can substitute white
or to taste	potato)
1 to 4 tablespoons + 3 cups	Chopped cilantro (optional)
water	Extra lime wedges (optional)

1. In a large pot over medium-high heat, combine the vinegar, onion, bell peppers, salt, black pepper, cumin seeds, oregano, allspice, and red-pepper flakes. Cook for 5 to 7 minutes, or until the onions and red peppers start to soften. Add 1 to 2 tablespoons of water if needed to keep the vegetables from sticking. Add the garlic and stir. Cover, reduce the heat to medium, and cook for another few minutes, until the garlic is softened. If anything is sticking or burning, add another 1 to 2 tablespoons of water. When the garlic is soft, add the tomato paste, lime juice, ½ teaspoon of the syrup, 3½ cups of the beans, and the remaining 3 cups water. Use an immersion blender to puree the soup until it's fairly smooth. Add the bay leaf and sweet potato, increase the heat to high to bring to a boil, then reduce the heat to low and simmer for 20 to 30 minutes. Add the remaining 1 cup black beans. Taste, and add the remaining ½ teaspoon syrup, if desired. Stir, simmer for another few minutes, then serve, seasoning to taste and topping with the cilantro (if using) and lime wedges (if using).

Per Serving:

calorie: 368 | fat: 2g | protein: 19g | carbs: 73g | sugars: 10g | fiber: 24g | sodium: 1049mg

Spanish Black Bean Soup

Prep time: 5 minutes | Cook time: 1 hour 10 minutes

| Serves 6

1½ cups plus 2 teaspoons low-	1 teaspoon cumin
sodium chicken broth, divided	1 teaspoon chili powder or ½
1 teaspoon extra-virgin olive oil	teaspoon cayenne pepper
3 garlic cloves, minced	1 red bell pepper, chopped
1 yellow onion, minced	1 carrot, coarsely chopped
1 teaspoon minced fresh	3 cups cooked black beans
oregano	½ cup dry red wine

1. In a large pot, heat 2 teaspoons of the chicken broth and the olive oil. Add the garlic and onion, and sauté for 3 minutes. Add

the oregano, cumin, and chili powder; stir for another minute. Add the red pepper and carrot. 2. Puree 1½ cups of the black beans in a blender or food processor. Add the pureed beans, the remaining 1½ cups of whole black beans, the remaining 1½ cups of chicken broth, and the red wine to the stockpot. Simmer 1 hour. 3. Taste before serving; add additional spices if you like.

Per Serving:

calories: 160 | fat: 3g | protein: 9g | carbs: 25g | sugars: 1g | fiber: 8g | sodium: 48mg

Nancy's Vegetable Beef Soup

Prep time: 25 minutes | Cook time: 8 hours | Serves 8

2 pounds roast, cubed, or 2	stewed tomatoes
pounds stewing meat	5 teaspoons salt-free beef
15 ounces can corn	bouillon powder
15 ounces can green beans	Tabasco, to taste
1 pound bag frozen peas	½ teaspoons salt
40 ounces can no-added-salt	

1. Combine all ingredients in the Instant Pot. Do not drain vegetables. 2. Add water to fill inner pot only to the fill line. 3. Secure the lid, or use the glass lid and set the Instant Pot on Slow Cook mode, Low for 8 hours, or until meat is tender and vegetables are soft.

Per Serving:

calories: 229 | fat: 5g | protein: 23g | carbs: 24g | sugars: 10g | fiber: 6g | sodium: 545mg

Kickin' Chili

Prep time: 10 minutes | Cook time: 45 minutes |

Serves 2

1 tablespoon extra-virgin olive	1 (15 ounces) can pinto beans,
oil	drained and rinsed
½ cup chopped onions	2 cups water
1 garlic clove, minced	2 teaspoons ground cumin
1 celery stalk, chopped	2 teaspoons chili powder
½ cup chopped bell peppers,	½ teaspoon cayenne pepper
any color	Salt, to season
1 cup diced tomatoes, undrained	Freshly ground black pepper, to
1 cup frozen broccoli florets	season

1. In a large pot set over medium heat, heat the olive oil. 2. Add the onions. Cook for about 5 minutes, or until tender. 3. Add the garlic. Cook for 2 to 3 minutes, or until lightly browned. 4. Add the celery and bell peppers. Cook for 5 minutes, or until the vegetables are soft. 5. Stir in the tomatoes, broccoli, pinto beans, and water. 6. Add the cumin, chili powder, and cayenne pepper. Season with salt and pepper. Stir to combine. Simmer for 30 minutes, stirring frequently. 7. Serve hot and enjoy!

Per Serving:

calories: 249 | fat: 5g | protein: 14g | carbs: 42g | sugars: 6g | fiber: 13g | sodium: 739mg

Chapter 11 Desserts

Strawberry Cheesecake in a Jar

Prep time: 5 minutes | Cook time: 0 minutes | Serves 8

½ cup (55 g) raw cashews
¼ cup (60 g) all-natural peanut butter
2 tablespoons (12 g) almond flour
1 large pitted Medjool date
1 cup (200 g) coarsely chopped strawberries, plus more as needed

8 ounces (227 g) cream cheese
½ cup (100 g) plain nonfat Greek yogurt
¼ cup (60 ml) pure maple syrup
Zest of 1 medium lemon, plus more as needed
1 tablespoon (15 ml) pure vanilla extract

1. In a food processor, combine the cashews, peanut butter, almond flour, and Medjool date. Process the ingredients until a dough forms. 2. Divide the dough among eight (8 ounces [227 ml]) mason jars. Press the dough down into each jar to make a crust. 3. Divide the strawberries among the jars on top of the crusts. 4. In a food processor or high-power blender, combine the cream cheese, yogurt, maple syrup, lemon zest, and vanilla. Process the ingredients until they are smooth. 5. Divide the cheesecake mixture evenly among the jars, tapping them gently on the counter to shake out all the air bubbles. 6. Top the cheesecakes with additional strawberries and lemon zest if desired. 7. Refrigerate the cheesecakes for at least 2 hours or overnight before serving.

Per Serving:
calorie: 253 | fat: 18g | protein: 7g | carbs: 17g | sugars: 12g | fiber: 2g | sodium: 115mg

Crustless Key Lime Cheesecake

Prep time: 15 minutes | Cook time: 35 minutes | Serves 8

Nonstick cooking spray
16 ounces light cream cheese (Neufchâtel), softened
⅔ cup granulated erythritol sweetener
¼ cup unsweetened Key lime juice (I like Nellie & Joe's

Famous Key West Lime Juice)
½ teaspoon vanilla extract
¼ cup plain Greek yogurt
1 teaspoon grated lime zest
2 large eggs
Whipped cream, for garnish (optional)

1. Spray a 7-inch springform pan with nonstick cooking spray. Line the bottom and partway up the sides of the pan with foil. 2. Put the cream cheese in a large bowl. Use an electric mixer to whip the cream cheese until smooth, about 2 minutes. Add the erythritol, lime juice, vanilla, yogurt, and zest, and blend until smooth. Stop the mixer and scrape down the sides of the bowl with a rubber spatula. With the mixer on low speed, add the eggs, one at a time, blending until just mixed. (Don't overbeat the eggs.) 3. Pour the mixture into the prepared pan. Drape a paper towel over the top of the pan, not touching the cream cheese mixture, and tightly wrap the top of the pan in foil. (Your goal here is to keep out as much moisture as possible.) 4. Pour 1 cup of water into the electric pressure cooker. 5. Place the foil-covered pan onto the wire rack and carefully lower it into the pot. 6. Close and lock the lid of the pressure cooker. Set the valve to sealing. 7. Cook on high pressure for 35 minutes. 8. When the cooking is complete, hit Cancel. Allow the pressure to release naturally for 20 minutes, then quick release any remaining pressure. 9. Once the pin drops, unlock and remove the lid. 10. Using the handles of the wire rack, carefully transfer the pan to a cooling rack. Cool to room temperature, then refrigerate for at least 3 hours. 11. When ready to serve, run a thin rubber spatula around the rim of the cheesecake to loosen it, then remove the ring. 12. Slice into wedges and serve with whipped cream (if using).

Per Serving:
calories: 127 | fat: 2g | protein: 11g | carbs: 17g | sugars: 14g | fiber: 0g | sodium: 423mg

Strawberry Cream Cheese Crepes

Prep time: 10 minutes | Cook time: 10 minutes | Serves 4

½ cup old-fashioned oats
1 cup unsweetened plain almond milk
1 egg
3 teaspoons honey, divided

Nonstick cooking spray
2 ounces low-fat cream cheese
¼ cup low-fat cottage cheese
2 cups sliced strawberries

1. In a blender jar, process the oats until they resemble flour. Add the almond milk, egg, and 1½ teaspoons honey, and process until smooth. 2. Heat a large skillet over medium heat. Spray with nonstick cooking spray to coat. 3. Add ¼ cup of oat batter to the pan and quickly swirl around to coat the bottom of the pan and let cook for 2 to 3 minutes. When the edges begin to turn brown, flip the crepe with a spatula and cook until lightly browned and firm, about 1 minute. Transfer to a plate. Continue with the remaining batter, spraying the skillet with nonstick cooking spray before adding more batter. Set the cooked crepes aside, loosely covered with aluminum foil, while you make the filling. 4. Clean the blender jar, then combine the cream cheese, cottage cheese, and remaining 1½ teaspoons honey, and process until smooth. 5. Fill each crepe with 2 tablespoons of the cream cheese mixture, topped with ¼ cup of strawberries. Serve.

Per Serving:
calories: 149 | fat: 6g | protein: 6g | carbs: 20g | sugars: 10g | fiber: 3g | sodium: 177mg

Chocolate Baked Bananas

Prep time: 10 minutes | Cook time: 8 to 10 minutes |
Serves 5

4 to 5 large ripe bananas, sliced lengthwise
2 tablespoons coconut nectar or pure maple syrup
1 tablespoon cocoa powder
Couple pinches sea salt

2 tablespoons nondairy chocolate chips (for finishing)
1 tablespoon chopped pecans, walnuts, almonds, or pumpkin seeds (for finishing)

1. Line a baking sheet with parchment paper and preheat oven to 450°F. Place bananas on the parchment. In a bowl, mix the coconut nectar or maple syrup with the cocoa powder and salt. Stir well to fully combine. Drizzle the chocolate mixture over the bananas. Bake for 8 to 10 minutes, until bananas are softened and caramelized. Sprinkle on chocolate chips and nuts, and serve.

Per Serving:

calorie: 146 | fat: 3g | protein: 2g | carbs: 34g | sugars: 18g | fiber: 4g | sodium: 119mg

Pomegranate–Tequila Sunrise Jelly Shots

Prep time: 30 minutes | Cook time: 10 minutes |
Serves 12

¾ cup pulp-free orange juice
2 envelopes unflavored gelatin
6 tablespoons silver or gold tequila
½ cup 100% pomegranate juice

¼ cup sugar
¼ cup water
Whole orange slices or orange slice wedges

1. Lightly spray 12 (2 ounces) shot glasses with cooking spray; gently wipe any excess with paper towel. In 1-quart saucepan, pour orange juice; sprinkle 1 envelope gelatin evenly over juice to soften. Heat over low heat, stirring constantly, until gelatin is completely dissolved; remove from heat. Stir in tequila. Divide orange juice mixture evenly among shot glasses (about 2 tablespoons per glass). In 9-inch square pan, place shot glasses. Refrigerate 30 minutes or until almost set. 2. Meanwhile, in same saucepan, combine pomegranate juice, sugar and water. Sprinkle remaining 1 envelope gelatin evenly over juice to soften. Heat over low heat, stirring constantly, until gelatin is completely dissolved; remove from heat. 3. Remove shot glasses from refrigerator (orange layer should appear mostly set). Pour pomegranate mixture evenly over top of orange layer in glasses (about 4 teaspoons per glass). Refrigerate at least 3 hours until completely chilled and firm. 4. Just before serving, dip a table knife in hot water; slide knife along inside edge of shot glass to loosen. Shake jelly shot out of glass onto plate; repeat with remaining jelly shots. Serve each jelly shot on top of whole orange slice or serve jelly shots with orange slice wedges.

Per Serving:

calorie: 60 | fat: 0g | protein: 1g | carbs: 9g | sugars: 9g | fiber: 0g | sodium: 0mg

Simple Bread Pudding

Prep time: 25 minutes | Cook time: 40 minutes |
Serves 8

6 to 8 slices bread, cubed
2 cups fat-free milk
2 eggs
¼ cup sugar
1 teaspoon ground cinnamon
1 teaspoon vanilla

1½ cups water
Sauce:
1 tablespoon cornstarch
6 ounces can concentrated grape juice

1. Place bread cubes in greased 1.6-quart baking dish. 2. Beat together milk and eggs. Stir in sugar, cinnamon and vanilla. Pour over bread and stir. 3. Cover with foil. 4. Place the trivet into your Instant Pot and pour in 1½ cup of water. Place a foil sling on top of the trivet, then place the baking dish on top. 5. Secure the lid and make sure lid is set to sealing. Press Manual and set time for 30 minutes. 6. When cook time is up, let the pressure release naturally for 15 minutes, then release any remaining pressure manually. Carefully remove the springform pan by using hot pads to lift the baking dish out by the foil sling. Let sit for a few minutes, uncovered, while you make the sauce. 7. Combine cornstarch and concentrated juice in saucepan. Heat until boiling, stirring constantly, until sauce is thickened. Serve drizzled over bread pudding.

Per Serving:

calories: 179 | fat: 2g | protein: 5g | carbs: 35g | sugars: 24g | fiber: 1g | sodium: 153mg

Orange Praline with Yogurt

Prep time: 10 minutes | Cook time: 10 minutes |
Serves 6

3 tablespoons sugar
4 teaspoons water
⅓ cup slivered almonds, toasted
½ teaspoon ground cinnamon
⅛ teaspoon ground cloves

1 tablespoon orange zest (optional)
Pinch kosher salt
3 cups plain Greek yogurt

1. Preheat the oven to 375°F. Line a baking sheet with parchment paper. 2. In a small saucepan, stir together the sugar and water and cook over high heat until light golden-brown in color, 3 to 4 minutes. Do not stir, but instead gently swirl to help the sugar dissolve. Add the almonds and cook for 1 minute. The goal is to coat the almonds with the heated sugar (think caramel here) without burning. Pour the mixture onto the prepared baking sheet and set aside to cool for about 5 minutes. 3. Meanwhile, in a medium bowl, stir together the cinnamon, cloves, orange zest (if using), and salt. 4. Break the praline into smaller pieces and toss them in the spices. 5. Evenly divide the yogurt among six bowls and serve topped with the spiced praline. Store the praline in a sealed container at room temperature for up to 2 weeks.

Per Serving:

calories: 126 | fat: 3g | protein: 8g | carbs: 16g | sugars: 15g | fiber: 1g | sodium: 250mg

Chewy Chocolate-Oat Bars

Prep time: 20 minutes | Cook time: 30 minutes |
Makes 16 bars

¾ cup semisweet chocolate chips
⅓ cup fat-free sweetened condensed milk (from 14-oz can)
1 cup whole wheat flour
½ cup quick-cooking oats
½ teaspoon baking powder
½ teaspoon baking soda
¼ teaspoon salt

¼ cup fat-free egg product or 1 egg
¾ cup packed brown sugar
¼ cup canola oil
1 teaspoon vanilla
2 tablespoons quick-cooking oats
2 teaspoons butter or margarine, softened

1 Heat oven to 350°F. Spray 8-inch or 9-inch square pan with cooking spray. 2 In 1-quart saucepan, heat chocolate chips and milk over low heat, stirring frequently, until chocolate is melted and mixture is smooth. Remove from heat. 3 In large bowl, mix flour, ½ cup oats, the baking powder, baking soda and salt; set aside. In medium bowl, stir egg product, brown sugar, oil and vanilla with fork until smooth. Stir into flour mixture until blended. Reserve ½ cup dough in small bowl for topping. 4 Pat remaining dough in pan (if dough is sticky, spray fingers with cooking spray or dust with flour). Spread chocolate mixture over dough. Add 2 tablespoons oats and the butter to reserved ½ cup dough; mix with pastry blender or fork until well mixed. Place small pieces of mixture evenly over chocolate mixture. 5 Bake 20 to 25 minutes or until top is golden and firm. Cool completely, about 1 hour 30 minutes. For bars, cut into 4 rows by 4 rows.

Per Serving:

1 Bar: calorie: 180 | fat: 7g | protein: 3g | carbs: 27g | sugars: 18g | fiber: 1g | sodium: 115mg

Mango Nice Cream

Prep time: 10 minutes | Cook time: 0 minutes |
Serves 4

2 cups frozen mango chunks
1 cup frozen, sliced, overripe banana (can use room temperature, but must be overripe)
Pinch of sea salt

½ teaspoon pure vanilla extract
¼ cup + 1 to 2 tablespoons low-fat nondairy milk
2 to 3 tablespoons coconut nectar or pure maple syrup (optional)

1. In a food processor or high-speed blender, combine the mango, banana, salt, vanilla, and ¼ cup of the milk. Pulse to get things moving, and then puree, adding the remaining 1 to 2 tablespoons milk if needed. Taste, and add the nectar or syrup, if desired. Serve, or transfer to an airtight container and freeze for an hour or more to set more firmly before serving.

Per Serving:

calorie: 116 | fat: 0.5g | protein: 1g | carbs: 29g | sugars: 22g | fiber: 2g | sodium: 81mg

Chipotle Black Bean Brownies

Prep time: 15 minutes | Cook time: 30 minutes |
Serves 8

Nonstick cooking spray
½ cup dark chocolate chips, divided
¾ cup cooked calypso beans or black beans
½ cup extra-virgin olive oil
2 large eggs
¼ cup unsweetened dark chocolate cocoa powder

⅓ cup honey
1 teaspoon vanilla extract
⅓ cup white wheat flour
½ teaspoon chipotle chili powder
½ teaspoon ground cinnamon
½ teaspoon baking powder
½ teaspoon kosher salt

1. Spray a 7-inch Bundt pan with nonstick cooking spray. 2. Place half of the chocolate chips in a small bowl and microwave them for 30 seconds. Stir and repeat, if necessary, until the chips have completely melted. 3. In a food processor, blend the beans and oil together. Add the melted chocolate chips, eggs, cocoa powder, honey, and vanilla. Blend until the mixture is smooth. 4. In a large bowl, whisk together the flour, chili powder, cinnamon, baking powder, and salt. Pour the bean mixture from the food processor into the bowl and stir with a wooden spoon until well combined. Stir in the remaining chocolate chips. 5. Pour the batter into the prepared Bundt pan. Cover loosely with foil. 6. Pour 1 cup of water into the electric pressure cooker. 7. Place the Bundt pan onto the wire rack and lower it into the pressure cooker. 8. Close and lock the lid of the pressure cooker. Set the valve to sealing. 9. Cook on high pressure for 30 minutes. 10. When the cooking is complete, hit Cancel and quick release the pressure. 11. Once the pin drops, unlock and remove the lid. 12. Carefully transfer the pan to a cooling rack for about 10 minutes, then invert the cake onto the rack and let it cool completely. 13. Cut into slices and serve.

Per Serving:

(1 slice): calories: 296 | fat: 20g | protein: 5g | carbs: 29g | sugars: 16g | fiber: 4g | sodium: 224mg

Frozen Mocha Milkshake

Prep time: 5 minutes | Cook time: 0 minutes | Serves 1

1 cup (240 ml) unsweetened vanilla almond milk
3 tablespoons (18 g) unsweetened cocoa powder
2 teaspoons (4 g) instant espresso powder

1½ cups (210 g) crushed ice
½ medium avocado, peeled and pitted
1 tablespoon (15 ml) pure maple syrup
1 teaspoon pure vanilla extract

1. In a blender, combine the almond milk, cocoa powder, espresso powder, ice, avocado, maple syrup, and vanilla. Blend the ingredients on high speed for 60 seconds, until the milkshake is smooth.

Per Serving:

calorie: 307 | fat: 20g | protein: 6g | carbs: 33g | sugars: 13g | fiber: 13g | sodium: 173mg

Broiled Pineapple

Prep time: 5 minutes | Cook time: 5 minutes | Serves 4

4 large slices fresh pineapple
2 tablespoons canned coconut milk

2 tablespoons unsweetened shredded coconut
¼ teaspoon sea salt

1. Preheat the oven broiler on high. 2. On a rimmed baking sheet, arrange the pineapple in a single layer. Brush lightly with the coconut milk and sprinkle with the coconut. 3. Broil until the pineapple begins to brown, 3 to 5 minutes. 4. Sprinkle with the sea salt.

Per Serving:

calories: 110 | fat: 3g | protein: 1g | carbs: 23g | sugars: 15g | fiber: 3g | sodium: 16mg

Walnut Macaroons

Prep time: 30 minutes | Cook time: 15 minutes | Serves 14

2 cups quick-cooking oats
¼ cup dried organic unsweetened coconut
2 tablespoons granulated sugar substitute (such as stevia)

2 teaspoons vanilla extract
½ cup canola oil
¼ cup egg whites, beaten until stiff
½ cup finely chopped walnuts

1. In a medium bowl, combine the oats, coconut, sugar substitute, vanilla, and oil; mix thoroughly. Cover, and refrigerate overnight. 2. Preheat the oven to 350 degrees. Carefully fold the egg whites and walnuts into the mixture; blend thoroughly. 3. Pack the cookie mixture into a teaspoon, level, and push out onto ungreased cookie sheets. 4. Bake the cookies at 350 degrees for 15 minutes or until the tops are golden brown. Transfer the cookies to racks, and cool.

Per Serving:

calories: 184 | fat: 12g | protein: 5g | carbs: 16g | sugars: 0g | fiber: 3g | sodium: 9mg

Avocado Chocolate Mousse

Prep time: 5 minutes | Cook time: 0 minutes | Serves 4

2 avocados, mashed
¼ cup canned coconut milk
2 tablespoons unsweetened cocoa powder

2 tablespoons pure maple syrup
½ teaspoon espresso powder
½ teaspoon vanilla extract

1. In a blender, combine all of the ingredients. Blend until smooth. 2. Pour the mixture into 4 small bowls and serve.

Per Serving:

calories: 222 | fat: 18g | protein: 3g | carbs: 17g | sugars: 7g | fiber: 8g | sodium: 11mg

Double-Ginger Cookies

Prep time: 45 minutes | Cook time: 8 to 10 minutes | Makes 5 dozen cookies

¾ cup sugar
¼ cup butter or margarine, softened
1 egg or ¼ cup fat-free egg product
¼ cup molasses
1¾ cups all-purpose flour
1 teaspoon baking soda

½ teaspoon ground cinnamon
½ teaspoon ground ginger
¼ teaspoon ground cloves
¼ teaspoon salt
¼ cup sugar
¼ cup orange marmalade
2 tablespoons finely chopped crystallized ginger

1. In medium bowl, beat ¾ cup sugar, the butter, egg and molasses with electric mixer on medium speed, or mix with spoon. Stir in flour, baking soda, cinnamon, ground ginger, cloves and salt. Cover and refrigerate at least 2 hours, until firm. 2. Heat oven to 350°F. Lightly spray cookie sheets with cooking spray. Place ¼ cup sugar in small bowl. Shape dough into ¾-inch balls; roll in sugar. Place balls about 2 inches apart on cookie sheet. Make indentation in center of each ball, using finger. Fill each indentation with slightly less than ¼ teaspoon of the marmalade. Sprinkle with crystallized ginger. 3. Bake 8 to 10 minutes or until set. Immediately transfer from cookie sheets to cooling racks. Cool completely, about 30 minutes.

Per Serving:

1 Cookie: calorie: 45 | fat: 1g | protein: 0g | carbs: 9g | sugars: 5g | fiber: 0g | sodium: 40mg

Oatmeal Cookies

Prep time: 5 minutes | Cook time: 15 minutes | Serves 16

¾ cup almond flour
¾ cup old-fashioned oats
¼ cup shredded unsweetened coconut
1 teaspoon baking powder
1 teaspoon ground cinnamon

¼ teaspoon salt
¼ cup unsweetened applesauce
1 large egg
1 tablespoon pure maple syrup
2 tablespoons coconut oil, melted

1. Preheat the oven to 350°F. 2. In a medium mixing bowl, combine the almond flour, oats, coconut, baking powder, cinnamon, and salt, and mix well. 3. In another medium bowl, combine the applesauce, egg, maple syrup, and coconut oil, and mix. Stir the wet mixture into the dry mixture. 4. Form the dough into balls a little bigger than a tablespoon and place on a baking sheet, leaving at least 1 inch between them. Bake for 12 minutes until the cookies are just browned. Remove from the oven and let cool for 5 minutes. 5. Using a spatula, remove the cookies and cool on a rack.

Per Serving:

calorie: 76 | fat: 6g | protein: 2g | carbs: 5g | sugars: 1g | fiber: 1g | sodium: 57mg

Grilled Watermelon with Avocado Mousse

Prep time: 10 minutes | Cook time: 10 minutes | Serves 8

1 small, seedless watermelon, halved and cut into 1-inch rounds
2 ripe avocados, pitted and

peeled
½ cup fat-free plain yogurt
¼ teaspoon cayenne pepper

1. On a hot grill, grill the watermelon slices for 2 to 3 minutes on each side, or until you can see the grill marks. 2. To make the avocado mousse, in a blender, combine the avocados, yogurt, and cayenne and process until smooth. 3. To serve, cut each watermelon round in half. Top each with a generous dollop of avocado mousse.

Per Serving:

calories: 162 | fat: 8g | protein: 3g | carbs: 22g | sugars: 14g | fiber: 5g | sodium: 13mg

No-Bake Chocolate Peanut Butter Cookies

Prep time: 10 minutes | Cook time: 0 minutes | Makes 12 Cookies

¾ cup unsweetened shredded coconut
½ cup peanut butter
2 tablespoons cream cheese, at room temperature
2 tablespoons unsalted butter,

melted
2 tablespoons unsweetened cocoa powder
2 tablespoons pure maple syrup
½ teaspoon vanilla extract

1. In a medium bowl, mix all of the ingredients until well combined. 2. Spoon into 12 cookies on a platter lined with parchment paper. Refrigerate to set, about 2 hours.

Per Serving:

1 cookie: calories: 113 | fat: 9g | protein: 3g | carbs: 6g | sugars: 4g | fiber: 1g | sodium: 25mg

Pineapple Pear Medley

Prep time: 10 minutes | Cook time: 10 minutes | Serves 12

1 large orange
15 ounces canned unsweetened pineapple chunks, undrained
32 ounces canned unsweetened pear halves, drained

16 ounces canned unsweetened apricot halves, drained
6 whole cloves
2 cinnamon sticks

1. Peel the orange, and reserve the rind. Divide the orange into sections, and remove the membrane. 2. Drain the pineapple, reserve the juice, and set aside. 3. In a large bowl, combine the orange sections, pineapple, pears, and apricots. Toss, and set aside. 4. In a small saucepan over medium heat, combine the orange rind, pineapple juice, cloves, and cinnamon. Let simmer for 5–10 minutes; then strain the juices, and pour over the fruit. 5. Cover, and refrigerate for at least 2–3 hours. Toss before serving.

Per Serving:

calories: 67 | fat: 0g | protein: 1g | carbs: 67g | sugars: 11g | fiber: 4g | sodium: 2mg

Cream Cheese Swirl Brownies

Prep time: 10 minutes | Cook time: 20 minutes | Serves 12

2 eggs
¼ cup unsweetened applesauce
¼ cup coconut oil, melted
3 tablespoons pure maple syrup, divided
¼ cup unsweetened cocoa

powder
¼ cup coconut flour
¼ teaspoon salt
1 teaspoon baking powder
2 tablespoons low-fat cream cheese

1. Preheat the oven to 350°F. Grease an 8-by-8-inch baking dish. 2. In a large mixing bowl, beat the eggs with the applesauce, coconut oil, and 2 tablespoons of maple syrup. 3. Stir in the cocoa powder and coconut flour, and mix well. Sprinkle the salt and baking powder evenly over the surface and mix well to incorporate. Transfer the mixture to the prepared baking dish. 4. In a small, microwave-safe bowl, microwave the cream cheese for 10 to 20 seconds until softened. Add the remaining 1 tablespoon of maple syrup and mix to combine. 5. Drop the cream cheese onto the batter, and use a toothpick or chopstick to swirl it on the surface. Bake for 20 minutes, until a toothpick inserted in the center comes out clean. Cool and cut into 12 squares. 6. Store refrigerated in a covered container for up to 5 days.

Per Serving:

calories: 84 | fat: 6g | protein: 2g | carbs: 6g | sugars: 4g | fiber: 2g | sodium: 93mg

Low-Fat Cream Cheese Frosting

Prep time: 5 minutes | Cook time: 0 minutes | Serves 8

3 cups fat-free ricotta cheese
1⅓ cups plain fat-free yogurt, strained overnight in cheesecloth over a bowl set in the refrigerator

2 cups low-fat cottage cheese
⅓ cup fructose
3 tablespoons evaporated fat-free milk

1. In a large bowl, combine all the ingredients; beat well with electric beaters until slightly stiff. 2. Place frosting in a covered container, and refrigerate until ready to use (this frosting can be refrigerated for up to 1 week).

Per Serving:

calories: 209 | fat: 7g | protein: 24g | carbs: 9g | sugars: 7g | fiber: 1g | sodium: 594mg

Creamy Pineapple-Pecan Dessert Squares

Prep time: 25 minutes | Cook time: 0 minutes |

Serves 18

¾ cup boiling water
1 package (4-serving size) lemon sugar-free gelatin
1 cup unsweetened pineapple juice
1½ cups graham cracker crumbs
½ cup sugar
¼ cup shredded coconut
¼ cup chopped pecans

3 tablespoons butter or margarine, melted
1 package (8 ounces) fat-free cream cheese
1 container (8 ounces) fat-free sour cream
1 can (8 ounces) crushed pineapple, undrained

1 In large bowl, pour boiling water over gelatin; stir about 2 minutes or until gelatin is completely dissolved. Stir in pineapple juice. Refrigerate about 30 minutes or until mixture is syrupy and just beginning to thicken. 2 Meanwhile, in 13x9-inch (3-quart) glass baking dish, toss cracker crumbs, ¼ cup of the sugar, the coconut, pecans and melted butter until well mixed. Reserve ½ cup crumb mixture for topping. Press remaining mixture in bottom of dish. 3 In medium bowl, beat cream cheese, sour cream and remaining ¼ cup sugar with electric mixer on medium speed until smooth; set aside. 4 Beat gelatin mixture with electric mixer on low speed until foamy; beat on high speed until light and fluffy (mixture will look like beaten egg whites). Beat in cream cheese mixture just until mixed. Gently stir in pineapple (with liquid). Pour into crust-lined dish; smooth top. Sprinkle reserved ½ cup crumb mixture over top. Refrigerate about 4 hours or until set. For servings, cut into 6 rows by 3 rows.

Per Serving:

calorie: 120 | fat: 4.5g | protein: 3g | carbs: 18g | sugars: 11g | fiber: 0g | sodium: 180mg

Ice Cream with Warm Strawberry Rhubarb Sauce

Prep time: 10 minutes | Cook time: 15 minutes |

Serves 4

1 cup sliced strawberries
1 cup chopped rhubarb
2 tablespoons water
1 tablespoon honey

½ teaspoon cinnamon
4 (¼-cup) scoops sugar-free vanilla ice cream

1. In a medium pot, combine the strawberries, rhubarb, water, honey, and cinnamon. Bring to a simmer on medium heat, stirring. Reduce the heat to medium-low. Simmer, stirring frequently, until the rhubarb is soft, about 15 minutes. Allow to cool slightly. 2. Place 1 scoop of ice cream into each of 4 bowls. Spoon the sauce over the ice cream.

Per Serving:

calories: 52 | fat: 1g | protein: 1g | carbs: 10g | sugars: 6g | fiber: 2g | sodium: 11mg

Chocolate Chip Banana Cake

Prep time: 15 minutes | Cook time: 25 minutes |

Serves 8

Nonstick cooking spray
3 ripe bananas
½ cup buttermilk
3 tablespoons honey
1 teaspoon vanilla extract
2 large eggs, lightly beaten
3 tablespoons extra-virgin olive oil

1½ cups whole wheat pastry flour
⅛ teaspoon ground nutmeg
1 teaspoon ground cinnamon
¼ teaspoon salt
1 teaspoon baking soda
⅓ cup dark chocolate chips

1. Spray a 7-inch Bundt pan with nonstick cooking spray. 2. In a large bowl, mash the bananas. Add the buttermilk, honey, vanilla, eggs, and olive oil, and mix well. 3. In a medium bowl, whisk together the flour, nutmeg, cinnamon, salt, and baking soda. 4. Add the flour mixture to the banana mixture and mix well. Stir in the chocolate chips. Pour the batter into the prepared Bundt pan. Cover the pan with foil. 5. Pour 1 cup of water into the electric pressure cooker. Place the pan on the wire rack and lower it into the pressure cooker. 6. Close and lock the lid of the pressure cooker. Set the valve to sealing. 7. Cook on high pressure for 25 minutes. 8. When the cooking is complete, hit Cancel and quick release the pressure. 9. Once the pin drops, unlock and remove the lid. 10. Carefully transfer the pan to a cooling rack, uncover, and let it cool for 10 minutes. 11. Invert the cake onto the rack and let it cool for about an hour. 12. Slice and serve the cake.

Per Serving:

(1 slice): calories: 261 | fat: 11g | protein: 6g | carbs: 39g | sugars: 16g | fiber: 4g | sodium: 239mg

Instant Pot Tapioca

Prep time: 10 minutes | Cook time: 7 minutes |

Serves 6

2 cups water
1 cup small pearl tapioca
½ cup sugar
4 eggs
½ cup evaporated skim milk

Sugar substitute to equal ¼ cup sugar
1 teaspoon vanilla
Fruit of choice, optional

1. Combine water and tapioca in Instant Pot. 2. Secure lid and make sure vent is set to sealing. Press Manual and set for 5 minutes. 3. Perform a quick release. Press Cancel, remove lid, and press Sauté. 4. Whisk together eggs and evaporated milk. SLOWLY add to the Instant Pot, stirring constantly so the eggs don't scramble. 5. Stir in the sugar substitute until it's dissolved, press Cancel, then stir in the vanilla. 6. Allow to cool thoroughly, then refrigerate at least 4 hours.

Per Serving:

calorie: 262 | fat: 3g | protein: 6g | carbs: 50g | sugars: 28g | fiber: 0g | sodium: 75mg

Banana Pineapple Freeze

Prep time: 30 minutes | Cook time: 0 minutes |

Serves 12

2 cups mashed ripe bananas
2 cups unsweetened orange juice
2 tablespoon fresh lemon juice

1 cup unsweetened crushed pineapple, undrained
½ teaspoon ground cinnamon

1. In a food processor, combine all ingredients, and process until smooth and creamy. 2. Pour the mixture into a 9-x-9-x-2-inch baking dish, and freeze overnight or until firm. Serve chilled.

Per Serving:

calories: 60 | fat: 0g | protein: 1g | carbs: 15g | sugars: 9g | fiber: 1g | sodium: 1mg

Ambrosia

Prep time: 10 minutes | Cook time: 0 minutes |

Serves 8

3 oranges, peeled, sectioned, and quartered
2 (4 ounces) cups diced peaches in water, drained

1 cup shredded, unsweetened coconut
1 (8 ounces) container fat-free crème fraîche

1. In a large mixing bowl, combine the oranges, peaches, coconut, and crème fraîche. Gently toss until well mixed. Cover and refrigerate overnight.

Per Serving:

calories: 111 | fat: 5g | protein: 2g | carbs: 12g | sugars: 8g | fiber: 3g | sodium: 7mg

Spiced Pear Applesauce

Prep time: 15 minutes | Cook time: 5 minutes |

Makes: 3½ cups

1 pound pears, peeled, cored, and sliced
2 teaspoons apple pie spice or

cinnamon
Pinch kosher salt
Juice of ½ small lemon

1. In the electric pressure cooker, combine the apples, pears, apple pie spice, salt, lemon juice, and ¼ cup of water. 2. Close and lock the lid of the pressure cooker. Set the valve to sealing. 3. Cook on high pressure for 5 minutes. 4. When the cooking is complete, hit Cancel and let the pressure release naturally. 5. Once the pin drops, unlock and remove the lid. 6. Mash the apples and pears with a potato masher to the consistency you like. 7. Serve warm, or cool to room temperature and refrigerate.

Per Serving:

(½ cup): calories: 108 | fat: 1g | protein: 1g | carbs: 29g | sugars: 20g | fiber: 6g | sodium: 15mg

Oatmeal Raisin Cookies

Prep time: 5 minutes | Cook time: 15 minutes |

Serves 6

3 cups rolled oats
1 cup whole-wheat flour
1 teaspoon baking soda
2 teaspoons cinnamon
½ cup raisins

¼ cup unsweetened applesauce
¼ cup agave nectar
½ cup egg substitute
½ cup plain fat-free yogurt
1 teaspoon vanilla

1. Preheat the oven to 350 degrees. 2. In a medium bowl, combine the oats, flour, baking soda, cinnamon, and raisins. 3. In a large bowl, beat the applesauce, agave nectar, egg substitute, yogurt, and vanilla until creamy. Slowly add the dry ingredients, and mix together. 4. Spray cookie sheets with nonstick cooking spray, and drop by teaspoonfuls onto the cookie sheets. Bake for 12–15 minutes at 350 degrees; transfer to racks, and cool.

Per Serving:

calories: 274 | fat: 4g | protein: 14g | carbs: 64g | sugars: 16g | fiber: 10g | sodium: 56mg

Cream Cheese Shortbread Cookies

Prep time: 30 minutes | Cook time: 20 minutes |

Makes 12 cookies

¼ cup coconut oil, melted
2 ounces (57 g) cream cheese, softened
½ cup granular erythritol

1 large egg, whisked
2 cups blanched finely ground almond flour
1 teaspoon almond extract

1. Combine all ingredients in a large bowl to form a firm ball. 2. Place dough on a sheet of plastic wrap and roll into a 12-inch-long log shape. Roll log in plastic wrap and place in refrigerator 30 minutes to chill. 3. Remove log from plastic and slice into twelve equal cookies. Cut two sheets of parchment paper to fit air fryer basket. Place six cookies on each ungreased sheet. Place one sheet with cookies into air fryer basket. Adjust the temperature to 320°F (160°C) and bake for 10 minutes, turning cookies halfway through cooking. They will be lightly golden when done. Repeat with remaining cookies. 4. Let cool 15 minutes before serving to avoid crumbling.

Per Serving:

1 cookie: calories: 154 | fat: 14g | protein: 4g | carbs: 4g | net carbs: 2g | fiber: 2g

Chapter 12 Salads

Chickpea "Tuna" Salad

Prep time: 15 minutes | Cook time: 0 minutes |

Serves 2

2 cups canned chickpeas, drained and rinsed
½ cup plain nonfat Greek yogurt
2 small celery stalks, chopped
1 small cucumber, chopped
½ cup chopped red onion
2 tablespoons freshly squeezed

lemon juice
1 tablespoon chia seeds
1 garlic clove, chopped
1 teaspoon minced fresh parsley
Salt, to season
Freshly ground black pepper, to season
2 large romaine lettuce leaves

1. In a medium bowl, roughly mash the chickpeas with the back of a fork. 2. Add the yogurt, celery, cucumber, red onion, lemon juice, chia seeds, garlic, and parsley. Mix well. Season with salt and pepper. 3. Place half of the chickpea mixture on each romaine lettuce leaf. Wrap and serve chilled or at room temperature.

Per Serving:

calorie: 293 | fat: 6g | protein: 17g | carbs: 46g | sugars: 14g | fiber: 13g | sodium: 401mg

Three Bean and Basil Salad

Prep time: 10 minutes | Cook time: 0 minutes |

Serves 8

1 (15 ounces) can low-sodium chickpeas, drained and rinsed
1 (15 ounces) can low-sodium kidney beans, drained and rinsed
1 (15 ounces) can low-sodium white beans, drained and rinsed
1 red bell pepper, seeded and finely chopped
¼ cup chopped scallions, both

white and green parts
¼ cup finely chopped fresh basil
3 garlic cloves, minced
2 tablespoons extra-virgin olive oil
1 tablespoon red wine vinegar
1 teaspoon Dijon mustard
¼ teaspoon freshly ground black pepper

1. In a large mixing bowl, combine the chickpeas, kidney beans, white beans, bell pepper, scallions, basil, and garlic. Toss gently to combine. 2. In a small bowl, combine the olive oil, vinegar, mustard, and pepper. Toss with the salad. 3. Cover and refrigerate for an hour before serving, to allow the flavors to mix.

Per Serving:

Calorie: 193 | fat: 5g | protein: 10g | carbs: 29g | sugars: 3g | fiber: 8g | sodium: 246mg

Cucumber-Mango Salad

Prep time: 20 minutes | Cook time: 0 minutes |

Serves 4

1 small cucumber
1 medium mango
¼ teaspoon grated lime peel
1 tablespoon lime juice

1 teaspoon honey
¼ teaspoon ground cumin
Pinch salt
4 leaves Bibb lettuce

1 Cut cucumber lengthwise in half; scoop out seeds. Chop cucumber (about 1 cup). 2 Score skin of mango lengthwise into fourths with knife; peel skin. Cut peeled mango lengthwise close to both sides of pit. Chop mango into ½-inch cubes. 3 In small bowl, mix lime peel, lime juice, honey, cumin and salt. Stir in cucumber and mango. Place lettuce leaves on serving plates. Spoon mango mixture onto lettuce leaves.

Per Serving:

calorie: 50 | fat: 0g | protein: 0g | carbs: 12g | sugars: 9g | fiber: 1g | sodium: 40mg

Grilled Romaine with White Beans

Prep time: 5 minutes | Cook time: 8 minutes | Serves

4 to 6

3 tablespoons extra-virgin olive oil, divided
2 large heads romaine lettuce, halved lengthwise
2 tablespoons white miso

1 tablespoon water, plus more as needed
1 (15 ounces) can white beans, rinsed and drained
½ cup chopped fresh parsley

1. Preheat the grill or a grill pan. 2. Drizzle 2 tablespoons of extra-virgin olive oil over the cut sides of the romaine lettuce. 3. In a medium bowl, whisk the remaining 1 tablespoon of extra-virgin olive oil with the white miso and about 1 tablespoon of water. Add more water, if necessary, to reach a thin consistency. Add the white beans and parsley to the bowl, stir, adjust the seasonings as desired, and set aside. 4. When the grill is hot, put the romaine on the grill and cook for 1 to 2 minutes on each side or until lightly charred with grill marks. Remove the lettuce from the grill and repeat with remaining lettuce halves. Set the lettuce aside on a platter or individual plates and top with the beans.

Per Serving:

calorie: 242 | fat: 10g | protein: 11g | carbs: 31g | sugars: 4g | fiber: 11g | sodium: 282mg

Roasted Carrot and Quinoa with Goat Cheese

Prep time: 10 minutes | Cook time: 20 minutes |

Serves 4

4 large carrots, cut into ⅛-inch-thick rounds
4 tablespoons oil (olive, safflower, or grapeseed), divided
2 teaspoons paprika
1 teaspoon turmeric

2 teaspoons ground cumin
2 cups water
1 cup quinoa, rinsed
½ cup shelled pistachios, toasted
4 ounces goat cheese
12 ounces salad greens

1. Preheat the oven to 400°F. Line a baking sheet with parchment paper. 2. In a large bowl, toss together the carrots, 2 tablespoons of oil, the paprika, turmeric, and cumin until the carrots are well coated. Spread them evenly on the prepared baking sheet and roast until tender, 15 to 17 minutes. 3. In a medium saucepan, combine the water and quinoa over high heat. Bring to a boil, reduce the heat to low and simmer until tender, about 15 minutes. 4. Transfer the roasted carrots to a large bowl and add the cooked quinoa, remaining 2 tablespoons of oil, the pistachios, and goat cheese and toss to combine. 5. Evenly divide the greens among four plates and top with the carrot mixture. Serve. 6. Store any leftovers in an airtight container in the refrigerator for up to 2 days.

Per Serving:

calorie: 544 | fat: 33g | protein: 21g | carbs: 43g | sugars: 6g | fiber: 9g | sodium: 202mg

Zucchini, Carrot, and Fennel Salad

Prep time: 10 minutes | Cook time: 8 minutes |

Serves ½ cup

2 medium carrots, peeled and julienned
1 medium zucchini, julienned
½ medium fennel bulb, core removed and julienned
1 tablespoon fresh orange juice
2 tablespoons Dijon mustard
3 tablespoons extra-virgin olive oil
1 teaspoon white wine vinegar

½ teaspoon dried thyme
1 tablespoon finely minced parsley
¼ teaspoon salt
¼ teaspoon freshly ground black pepper
¼ cup chopped walnuts
1 medium head romaine lettuce, washed and leaves separated

1. Place the carrots, zucchini, and fennel in a medium bowl; set aside. 2. In a medium bowl, combine the orange juice, mustard, olive oil, vinegar, thyme, parsley, salt, and pepper; mix well. 3. Pour the dressing over the vegetables and toss. Add the walnuts, and mix again. Refrigerate until ready to serve. 4. To serve, line a bowl or plates with lettuce leaves, and spoon ½ cup of salad on top.

Per Serving:

calorie: 201 | fat: 16g | protein: 5g | carbs: 14g | sugars: 6g | fiber: 6g | sodium: 285mg

Edamame and Walnut Salad

Prep time: 10 minutes | Cook time: 0 minutes |

Serves 2

For the vinaigrette
2 tablespoons balsamic vinegar
1 tablespoon extra-virgin olive oil
1 teaspoon grated fresh ginger
½ teaspoon Dijon mustard
Pinch salt
Freshly ground black pepper, to

season
For the salad
1 cup shelled edamame
½ cup shredded carrots
½ cup shredded red cabbage
½ cup walnut halves
6 cups prewashed baby spinach, divided

To make the vinaigrette In a small bowl, whisk together the balsamic vinegar, olive oil, ginger, Dijon mustard, and salt. Season with pepper. Set aside. To make the salad 1. In a medium bowl, mix together the edamame, carrots, red cabbage, and walnuts. 2. Add the vinaigrette. Toss to coat. 3. Place 3 cups of spinach on each of 2 serving plates. 4. Top each serving with half of the dressed vegetables. 5. Enjoy immediately!

Per Serving:

calorie: 341 | fat: 26g | protein: 13g | carbs: 19g | sugars: 7g | fiber: 8g | sodium: 117mg

Mediterranean Pasta Salad with Goat Cheese

Prep time: 25 minutes | Cook time: 0 minutes |

Serves 4

½ cup (75 g) grape tomatoes, sliced in half lengthwise
1 medium red bell pepper, coarsely chopped
½ medium red onion, sliced into thin strips
1 medium zucchini, coarsely chopped
1 cup (175 g) broccoli florets
½ cup (110 g) oil-packed artichoke hearts, drained
¼ cup (60 ml) olive oil

½ teaspoon sea salt
½ teaspoon black pepper
1 tablespoon (3 g) dried oregano
½ teaspoon garlic powder
4 ounces (113 g) crumbled goat cheese
½ cup (50 g) shaved Parmesan cheese
8 ounces (227 g) lentil or chickpea penne pasta, cooked, rinsed, and drained

1. In a large bowl, combine the tomatoes, bell pepper, onion, zucchini, broccoli, artichoke hearts, oil, sea salt, black pepper, oregano, garlic powder, goat cheese, and Parmesan cheese. Gently mix everything together to combine and coat all of the ingredients with the oil. 2. Add the pasta to the bowl and stir to combine. 3. Let the pasta salad rest for 1 to 2 hours in the refrigerator to marinate it, or serve the pasta salad immediately if desired.

Per Serving:

calorie: 477 | fat: 24g | protein: 23g | carbs: 41g | sugars: 6g | fiber: 6g | sodium: 706mg

Chicken, Spinach, and Berry Salad

Prep time: 5 minutes | Cook time: 0 minutes | Serves 4

For The Salad
8 cups baby spinach
2 cups shredded rotisserie chicken
½ cup sliced strawberries or
For The Dressing
2 tablespoons extra-virgin olive oil

other berries
½ cup sliced almonds
1 avocado, sliced
¼ cup crumbled feta (optional)

2 teaspoons honey
2 teaspoons balsamic vinegar

To Make The Salad 1. In a large bowl, combine the spinach, chicken, strawberries, and almonds. 2. Pour the dressing over the salad and lightly toss. 3. Divide into four equal portions and top each with sliced avocado and 1 tablespoon of crumbled feta (if using). To Make The Dressing 4. In a small bowl, whisk together the olive oil, honey, and balsamic vinegar.

Per Serving:

calorie: 341 | fat: 22g | protein: 26g | carbs: 14g | sugars: 5g | fiber: 7g | sodium: 99mg

Warm Barley and Squash Salad with Balsamic Vinaigrette

Prep time: 20 minutes | Cook time: 40 minutes | Serves 8

1 small butternut squash
3 teaspoons plus 2 tablespoons extra-virgin olive oil, divided
2 cups broccoli florets
1 cup pearl barley
1 cup toasted chopped walnuts
2 cups baby kale

½ red onion, sliced
2 tablespoons balsamic vinegar
2 garlic cloves, minced
½ teaspoon salt
¼ teaspoon freshly ground black pepper

1. Preheat the oven to 400°F. Line a baking sheet with parchment paper. 2. Peel and seed the squash, and cut it into dice. In a large bowl, toss the squash with 2 teaspoons of olive oil. Transfer to the prepared baking sheet and roast for 20 minutes. 3. While the squash is roasting, toss the broccoli in the same bowl with 1 teaspoon of olive oil. After 20 minutes, flip the squash and push it to one side of the baking sheet. Add the broccoli to the other side and continue to roast for 20 more minutes until tender. 4. While the veggies are roasting, in a medium pot, cover the barley with several inches of water. Bring to a boil, then reduce the heat, cover, and simmer for 30 minutes until tender. Drain and rinse. 5. Transfer the barley to a large bowl, and toss with the cooked squash and broccoli, walnuts, kale, and onion. 6. In a small bowl, mix the remaining 2 tablespoons of olive oil, balsamic vinegar, garlic, salt, and pepper. Toss the salad with the dressing and serve.

Per Serving:

calories: 274 | fat: 15g | protein: 6g | carbs: 32g | sugars: 3g | fiber: 7g | sodium: 144mg

Celery and Apple Salad with Cider Vinaigrette

Prep time: 20 minutes | Cook time: 0 minutes | Serves 4

Dressing
2 tablespoons apple cider or apple juice
1 tablespoon cider vinegar
2 teaspoons canola oil
2 teaspoons finely chopped shallots
½ teaspoon Dijon mustard
½ teaspoon honey
½ teaspoon salt

Salad
2 cups chopped romaine lettuce
2 cups diagonally sliced celery
½ medium apple, unpeeled, sliced very thin (about 1 cup)
⅓ cup sweetened dried cranberries
2 tablespoons chopped walnuts
2 tablespoons crumbled blue cheese

1. In small bowl, beat all dressing ingredients with whisk until blended; set aside. 2. In medium bowl, place lettuce, celery, apple and cranberries; toss with dressing. To serve, arrange salad on 4 plates. Sprinkle with walnuts and blue cheese. Serve immediately.

Per Serving:

calorie: 130 | fat: 6g | protein: 2g | carbs: 17g | sugars: 13g | fiber: 3g | sodium: 410mg

Meatless Taco Salad

Prep time: 20 minutes | Cook time: 0 minutes | Serves 2

⅓ cup mashed avocado
¼ cup plain nonfat Greek yogurt
2 tablespoons chopped green bell pepper
1 tablespoon chopped scallions
1 tablespoon extra-virgin olive oil
⅛ teaspoon salt
¼ teaspoon chili powder
¼ teaspoon freshly ground

black pepper
½ teaspoon ground cumin
3 cups shredded romaine lettuce
8 cherry tomatoes, halved
1 cup canned kidney beans, rinsed and drained
¼ cup sliced black olives
½ cup crushed kale chips, divided
½ cup shredded nonfat Cheddar cheese, divided

1. In a small bowl, stir together the avocado, yogurt, green bell pepper, scallions, olive oil, salt, chili powder, pepper, and cumin. Set aside. 2. In a large bowl, mix the lettuce, tomatoes, kidney beans, and olives. 3. Evenly divide the lettuce mixture between 2 plates. 4. Top each with half of the avocado mixture. 5. Sprinkle each serving with ¼ cup of kale chips and ¼ cup of Cheddar cheese. 6. Enjoy immediately.

Per Serving:

calorie: 368 | fat: 21g | protein: 18g | carbs: 30g | sugars: 8g | fiber: 10g | sodium: 613mg

Chickpea Salad

Prep time: 15 minutes | Cook time: 0 minutes |
Serves 4

½ cup bottled balsamic vinaigrette
1 (15 ounces) can chickpeas, rinsed and drained
1 cup cherry tomatoes
1 small red onion, quartered and sliced
2 large cucumbers, peeled and
cut into bite-size pieces
1 large zucchini, cut into bite-size pieces
1 (10 ounces) package frozen shelled edamame, steamed or microwaved
Chopped fresh parsley, for garnish

1. Pour the vinaigrette into a large bowl. Add the chickpeas, tomatoes, onion, cucumbers, zucchini, and edamame and toss until all the ingredients are coated. 2. Garnish with chopped parsley.

Per Serving:
calorie: 188 | fat: 4g | protein: 10g | carbs: 29g | sugars: 11g | fiber: 8g | sodium: 171mg

Salmon Niçoise Salad

Prep time: 10 minutes | Cook time: 30 minutes |
Serves 1

salad
4 ounces (113 g) fresh salmon fillets
Cooking oil spray, as needed
1 teaspoon olive oil
Sea salt, as needed
Black pepper, as needed
2 cups (60 g) arugula
⅛ cup (17 g) assorted olives
½ cup (60 g) coarsely chopped

dressing
1 tablespoon (15 g) tahini
½ tablespoon (8 g) Dijon mustard
1 tablespoon (15 ml) fresh lemon juice

cucumber
1 large hard-boiled egg
½ cup (65 g) quartered baby potatoes
2 teaspoons (2 g) dried rosemary
2½ ounces (71 g) fresh green beans

3 tablespoons (45 ml) water
½ teaspoon dried dill
Sea salt, as needed
Black pepper, as needed

1. Preheat the oven to 400°F (204°C). Line a large baking sheet with parchment paper. 2. Bring a large pot of water to a boil over high heat. 3. To make the salad, heat a medium skillet over medium-high heat. Spray the salmon with the cooking oil spray and drizzle the oil on top. Place it in the skillet and cook for 2 to 3 minutes on each side (depending how thick the fillet is), until the outside is an opaque pink color and just barely starts to brown. Season the salmon with the salt and black pepper. 4. On a serving plate, arrange a bed of arugula. On the arugula, arrange the olives, cucumber, egg, and salmon. Set the plate aside. 5. Place the potatoes in a medium bowl. Add the rosemary and toss to coat the potatoes. Transfer them to the prepared baking sheet and bake them for 20 to 25 minutes, or until the potatoes are brown and crispy on the outside. 6. While the potatoes are roasting, prepare a large bowl of ice water. Add the green beans to the boiling water and cook them for 2 minutes. Quickly transfer the green beans to the bowl of ice water. Once they have cooled, add the green beans to the salad. 7. To make the dressing, mix together the tahini, mustard, lemon juice, water, dill, sea salt, and black pepper in a medium jar. 8. Add the potatoes to the salad, toss the salad with the dressing, and serve.

Per Serving:
calorie: 471 | fat: 23g | protein: 37g | carbs: 31g | sugars: 6g | fiber: 7g | sodium: 555mg

Winter Chicken and Citrus Salad

Prep time: 10 minutes | Cook time: 0 minutes |
Serves 4

4 cups baby spinach
2 tablespoons extra-virgin olive oil
1 tablespoon freshly squeezed lemon juice
⅛ teaspoon salt
Freshly ground black pepper
2 cups chopped cooked chicken
2 mandarin oranges, peeled and sectioned
½ peeled grapefruit, sectioned
¼ cup sliced almonds

1. In a large mixing bowl, toss the spinach with the olive oil, lemon juice, salt, and pepper. 2. Add the chicken, oranges, grapefruit, and almonds to the bowl. Toss gently. 3. Arrange on 4 plates and serve.

Per Serving:
calories: 249 | fat: 12g | protein: 24g | carbs: 11g | sugars: 7g | fiber: 3g | sodium: 135mg

Power Salad

Prep time: 15 minutes | Cook time: 0 minutes |
Serves 2

For the dressing
1 tablespoon extra-virgin olive oil
1 tablespoon freshly squeezed lemon juice
1 tablespoon balsamic vinegar
1 tablespoon chia seeds
1 teaspoon liquid stevia
Pinch salt
Freshly ground black pepper

For the salad
6 cups mixed baby greens
1 cup shelled edamame
1 cup chopped red cabbage
1 cup chopped red bell pepper
1 cup sliced fresh button mushrooms
½ cup sliced avocado
¼ cup sliced almonds
1 cup pea shoots, divided

To make the dressing 1. In a small bowl, whisk together the olive oil, lemon juice, balsamic vinegar, chia seeds, and stevia until well combined. Season with salt and pepper. To make the salad 2. In a large bowl, toss together the mixed greens, edamame, red cabbage, red bell pepper, mushrooms, avocado, and almonds. Drizzle the dressing over the salad. Toss again to coat well. 3. Divide the salad between 2 plates. Top each with ½ cup of pea shoots and serve.

Per Serving:
calorie: 449 | fat: 24g | protein: 22g | carbs: 47g | sugars: 11g | fiber: 16g | sodium: 86mg

Strawberry-Blueberry-Orange Salad

Prep time: 15 minutes | Cook time: 0 minutes |

Serves 8

¼ cup fat-free or reduced-fat mayonnaise
3 tablespoons sugar
1 tablespoon white vinegar
2 teaspoons poppy seed

2 cups fresh strawberry halves
2 cups fresh blueberries
1 orange, peeled, chopped
Sliced almonds, if desired

1 In small bowl, mix mayonnaise, sugar, vinegar and poppy seed with whisk until well blended. 2 In medium bowl, mix strawberries, blueberries and orange. Just before serving, pour dressing over fruit; toss. Sprinkle with almonds.

Per Serving:

calorie: 70 | fat: 1g | protein: 0g | carbs: 16g | sugars: 12g | fiber: 2g | sodium: 60mg

Quinoa, Beet, and Greens Salad

Prep time: 15 minutes | Cook time: 25 minutes |

Serves 2

For the vinaigrette
1 tablespoon extra-virgin olive oil
2 tablespoons red wine vinegar
1 garlic clove, chopped
Freshly ground black pepper, to season
For the salad
2 medium beets

1 small bunch fresh kale leaves, thoroughly washed, deveined, and dried
Extra-virgin olive oil cooking spray
⅓ cup dry quinoa
⅔ cup water
¼ cup chopped scallions
½ cup unsalted soy nuts

To make the vinaigrette In a large bowl, whisk together the olive oil, red wine vinegar, and garlic. Season with pepper. Set aside. To make the salad 1. Into a medium saucepan set over high heat, insert a steamer basket. Fill the pan with water to just below the bottom of the steamer. Cover and bring to a boil. 2. Add the beets. Cover and steam for 7 to 10 minutes, or until just tender. Remove from the steamer. Let sit until cool enough to handle. Peel and slice. Set aside. 3. Spray the kale leaves with cooking spray. Massage the leaves, breaking down the fibers so they're easier to chew. Chop finely. You should have 1 cup. 4. In a small saucepan set over high heat, mix together the quinoa and water. Bring to a boil. Reduce the heat to medium-low. Cover and simmer for about 15 minutes, or until the quinoa is tender and the liquid has been absorbed. Remove from the heat. 5. Immediately add half of the vinaigrette to the saucepan while fluffing the quinoa with a fork. Cover and refrigerate for at least 1 hour, or until completely cooled. Set aside the remaining vinaigrette. 6. Into the cooled quinoa, stir the chopped kale, scallions, soy nuts, sliced beets, and remaining vinaigrette. Toss lightly before serving.

Per Serving:

calorie: 461 | fat: 29g | protein: 14g | carbs: 41g | sugars: 7g | fiber: 9g | sodium: 100mg

Cheeseburger Wedge Salad

Prep time: 15 minutes | Cook time: 10 minutes |

Serves 4

salad
1 pound (454 g) lean ground beef
2 medium heads romaine lettuce, rinsed, dried, and sliced in half lengthwise
½ cup (60 g) shredded Cheddar cheese
½ cup (80 g) coarsely chopped tomatoes
⅓ cup (50 g) finely chopped red onion

1 small dill pickle, finely chopped (optional)
dressing
2 ounces (57 g) no-salt-added tomato paste
2 tablespoons (30 ml) apple cider vinegar
2 tablespoons (30 ml) water
1 tablespoon (15 ml) honey
¼ teaspoon sea salt
½ teaspoon onion powder
¼ teaspoon garlic powder

1. To make the salad, heat a large skillet over medium-high heat. Once the skillet is hot, add the beef and cook it for 9 to 10 minutes, until it is brown and cooked though. 2. Meanwhile, place a ½ head of romaine lettuce on each of four plates. Divide the beef evenly on top of each of the romaine halves. Then top each with the Cheddar cheese, tomatoes, onion, and pickle (if using). 3. To make the dressing, combine the tomato paste, vinegar, water, honey, sea salt, onion powder, and garlic powder in a small mason jar, secure the lid on top, and shake the jar thoroughly until everything is combined. Drizzle the dressing evenly over each salad and serve.

Per Serving:

calorie: 320 | fat: 14g | protein: 32g | carbs: 19g | sugars: 11g | fiber: 8g | sodium: 341mg

Three-Bean Salad with Black Bean Crumbles

Prep time: 15 minutes | Cook time: 0 minutes |

Serves 4

½ cup bottled Italian dressing
2 cups frozen black bean crumbles, microwaved per package instructions
1 cup cherry tomatoes, halved
1 (16 ounces) can or jar three-

bean salad mix, drained
1 medium onion, quartered and thinly sliced
4 cups romaine salad greens
1 cup shredded reduced-fat cheddar cheese, divided

1. Pour the Italian dressing into a large bowl. Add the black bean crumbles, cherry tomatoes, three-bean salad, and onion and mix until everything is well coated. 2. Divide the greens into 4 bowls and top each with the bean mixture. 3. Sprinkle ¼ cup of shredded cheddar cheese on each portion.

Per Serving:

calorie: 357 | fat: 10g | protein: 22g | carbs: 48g | sugars: 6g | fiber: 9g | sodium: 478mg

Shanghai Salad

Prep time: 5 minutes | Cook time: 10 minutes |

Serves 4

3 tablespoons canola oil	chestnuts, drained and sliced
1 teaspoon grated fresh ginger	6 scallions, cut into 2-inch
1 garlic clove, minced	pieces
8 ounces cooked lean flank	2 tablespoons dry sherry
steak, cut into 1-inch pieces	1 tablespoon light soy sauce
1½ cups fresh snow peas,	4 cups romaine lettuce,
trimmed	shredded
One 8-ounce can water	

1. In a large skillet, heat the oil over medium-high heat. Sauté the ginger, and garlic for 1 to 2 minutes. 2. Add the remaining ingredients (except the lettuce) to the skillet, and stir until heated through. 3. Arrange the shredded lettuce on a platter, spoon the mixture over the bed of lettuce, and serve.

Per Serving:

calorie: 242 | fat: 15g | protein: 16g | carbs: 12g | sugars: 5g | fiber: 4g | sodium: 236mg

Herbed Spring Peas

Prep time: 10 minutes | Cook time: 15 minutes |

Serves 6

1 tablespoon unsalted non-	vegetable broth
hydrogenated plant-based butter	3 cups fresh shelled peas
½ Vidalia onion, thinly sliced	1 tablespoon minced fresh
1 cup store-bought low-sodium	tarragon

1. In a skillet, melt the butter over medium heat. 2. Add the onion and sauté for 2 to 3 minutes, or until the onion is translucent. 3. Add the broth, and reduce the heat to low. 4. Add the peas and tarragon, cover, and cook for 7 to 10 minutes, or until the peas soften. 5. Serve.

Per Serving:

calorie: 43 | fat: 2g | protein: 2g | carbs: 6g | sugars: 3g | fiber: 2g | sodium: 159mg

Lentil Salad

Prep time: 10 minutes | Cook time: 45 minutes |

Serves 8

1 pound dried lentils, washed	oregano
(rinse with cold water in a	3 tablespoons fresh lemon juice
colander)	¼ teaspoon freshly ground
3 cups water	black pepper
2 tablespoons extra-virgin olive	2 large green bell peppers,
oil	cored, seeded, and diced
2 teaspoons cumin	2 large red bell peppers, cored,
1 teaspoon minced fresh	seeded, and diced

3 stalks celery, diced	1 red onion, minced

1. In a large saucepan over high heat, bring lentils and water to a boil. Reduce the heat to low, cover, and simmer for 35–45 minutes. Drain, and set aside. 2. In a large bowl, mix together the oil, cumin, oregano, lemon juice, and pepper until well blended. Add the lentils and the prepared vegetables. Cover, and chill in the refrigerator before serving.

Per Serving:

calorie: 261 | fat: 4g | protein: 15g | carbs: 43g | sugars: 5g | fiber: 8g | sodium: 15mg

Cabbage Slaw Salad

Prep time: 15 minutes | Cook time: 0 minutes |

Serves 6

2 cups finely chopped green	2 tablespoons extra-virgin olive
cabbage	oil
2 cups finely chopped red	2 tablespoons rice vinegar
cabbage	1 teaspoon honey
2 cups grated carrots	1 garlic clove, minced
3 scallions, both white and	¼ teaspoon salt
green parts, sliced	

1. In a large bowl, toss together the green and red cabbage, carrots, and scallions. 2. In a small bowl, whisk together the oil, vinegar, honey, garlic, and salt. 3. Pour the dressing over the veggies and mix to thoroughly combine. 4. Serve immediately, or cover and chill for several hours before serving.

Per Serving:

calories: 80 | fat: 5g | protein: 1g | carbs: 10g | sugars: 6g | fiber: 3g | sodium: 126mg

Herbed Tomato Salad

Prep time: 7 minutes | Cook time: 0 minutes | Serves

2 to 4

1 pint cherry tomatoes, halved	1 teaspoon sumac (optional)
1 bunch fresh parsley, leaves	2 tablespoons extra-virgin olive
only (stems discarded)	oil
1 cup cilantro, leaves only	Kosher salt
(stems discarded)	Freshly ground black pepper
¼ cup fresh dill	

1. In a medium bowl, carefully toss together the tomatoes, parsley, cilantro, dill, sumac (if using), extra-virgin olive oil, and salt and pepper to taste. 2. Store any leftovers in an airtight container in the refrigerator for up to 3 days, but the salad is best consumed on the day it is dressed.

Per Serving:

calorie: 113 | fat: 10g | protein: 2g | carbs: 7g | sugars: 3g | fiber: 3g | sodium: 30mg

Rainbow Quinoa Salad

Prep time: 10 minutes | Cook time: 0 minutes |

Serves 3

Dressing
3½ tablespoons orange juice
1 tablespoon apple cider vinegar
1 tablespoon pure maple syrup
1½ teaspoons yellow mustard
Couple pinches of cloves
Rounded ½ teaspoon sea salt
Freshly ground black pepper to taste
Salad
2 cups cooked quinoa, cooled

½ cup corn kernels
½ cup diced apple tossed in ½ teaspoon lemon juice
¼ cup diced red pepper
¼ cup sliced green onions or chives
1 can (15 ounces) black beans, rinsed and drained
Sea salt to taste
Freshly ground black pepper to taste

1. To make the dressing: In a large bowl, whisk together the orange juice, vinegar, syrup, mustard, cloves, salt, and pepper. 2. To make the salad: Add the quinoa, corn, apple, red pepper, green onion or chives, and black beans, and stir to combine well. Season with the salt and black pepper to taste. Serve, or store in an airtight container in the fridge.

Per Serving:

calorie: 355 | fat: 4g | protein: 15g | carbs: 68g | sugars: 12g | fiber: 15g | sodium: 955mg

Warm Sweet Potato and Black Bean Salad

Prep time: 5 minutes | Cook time: 35 minutes |

Serves 2

Extra-virgin olive oil cooking spray
1 large sweet potato, peeled and cubed
1 tablespoon extra-virgin olive oil
1 tablespoon balsamic vinegar
1 teaspoon dried rosemary

¼ teaspoon garlic powder
⅛ teaspoon salt
⅛ teaspoon freshly ground black pepper
1 cup canned black beans, drained and rinsed
2 tablespoons chopped chives

1. Preheat the oven to 450°F. 2. In a small baking dish coated with cooking spray, place the sweet potato cubes. Put the dish in the preheated oven. Bake for 20 to 35 minutes, uncovered, or until tender. 3. In a medium serving bowl, whisk together the olive oil, balsamic vinegar, rosemary, garlic powder, salt, and pepper. 4. Add the black beans and cooked sweet potato to the oil and herb mixture. Toss to coat. 5. Sprinkle with the chives. 6. Serve immediately and enjoy!

Per Serving:

calorie: 235 | fat: 7g | protein: 8g | carbs: 35g | sugars: 4g | fiber: 10g | sodium: 359mg

Romaine Lettuce Salad with Cranberry, Feta, and Beans

Prep time: 10 minutes | Cook time: 0 minutes |

Serves 2

1 cup chopped fresh green beans
6 cups washed and chopped romaine lettuce
1 cup sliced radishes
2 scallions, sliced
¼ cup chopped fresh oregano
1 cup canned kidney beans, drained and rinsed

½ cup cranberries, fresh or frozen
¼ cup crumbled fat-free feta cheese
1 tablespoon extra-virgin olive oil
Salt, to season
Freshly ground black pepper, to season

1. In a microwave-safe dish, add the green beans and a small amount of water. Microwave on high for about 2 minutes, or until tender. 2. In a large bowl, toss together the romaine lettuce, radishes, scallions, and oregano. 3. Add the green beans, kidney beans, cranberries, feta cheese, and olive oil. Season with salt and pepper. Toss to coat. 4. Evenly divide between 2 plates and enjoy immediately.

Per Serving:

calorie: 271 | fat: 9g | protein: 16g | carbs: 36g | sugars: 10g | fiber: 13g | sodium: 573mg

Thai Broccoli Slaw

Prep time: 20 minutes | Cook time: 0 minutes |

Serves 8

Dressing
2 tablespoons reduced-fat creamy peanut butter
1 tablespoon grated gingerroot
1 tablespoon rice vinegar
1 tablespoon orange marmalade
Slaw
3 cups broccoli slaw mix (from 10 ounces bag)
½ cup bite-size thin strips red bell pepper
½ cup julienne (matchstick-cut)

1½ teaspoons reduced-sodium soy sauce
¼ to ½ teaspoon chili garlic sauce

carrots
½ cup shredded red cabbage
2 tablespoons chopped fresh cilantro

1 In small bowl, combine all dressing ingredients. Beat with whisk, until blended. 2 In large bowl, toss all slaw ingredients. Pour dressing over slaw mixture; toss until coated. Cover and refrigerate at least 1 hour to blend flavors but no longer than 6 hours, tossing occasionally to blend dressing from bottom of bowl back into slaw mixture.

Per Serving:

calorie: 50 | fat: 1.5g | protein: 2g | carbs: 7g | sugars: 3g | fiber: 1g | sodium: 75mg

Shaved Brussels Sprouts and Kale with Poppy Seed Dressing

Prep time: 20 minutes | Cook time: 0 minutes |

Serves 4 to 6

1 pound Brussels sprouts, shaved	4 ounces shredded Romano cheese
1 bunch kale, thinly shredded	Poppy seed dressing
4 scallions, both white and green parts, thinly sliced	Kosher salt
	Freshly ground black pepper

1. In a large bowl, toss together the Brussels sprouts, kale, scallions, and Romano cheese. Add the dressing to the greens and toss to combine. Season with salt and pepper to taste.

Per Serving:

calorie: 139 | fat: 7g | protein: 11g | carbs: 11g | sugars: 3g | fiber: 4g | sodium: 357mg

Wild Rice Salad

Prep time: 5 minutes | Cook time: 45 minutes |

Serves 6

1 cup raw wild rice (rinsed)	¼ cup minced red bell pepper
4 cups cold water	1 shallot, minced
1 cup mandarin oranges, packed in their own juice (drain and reserve 2 tablespoons of liquid)	1 teaspoon minced thyme
	2 tablespoons raspberry vinegar
½ cup chopped celery	1 tablespoon extra-virgin olive oil

1. Place the rinsed, raw rice and the water in a saucepan. Bring to a boil, lower the heat, cover the pan, and cook for 45–50 minutes until the rice has absorbed the water. Set the rice aside to cool. 2. In a large bowl, combine the mandarin oranges, celery, red pepper, and shallot. 3. In a small bowl, combine the reserved juice, thyme, vinegar, and oil. 4. Add the rice to the mandarin oranges and vegetables. Pour the dressing over the salad, toss, and serve.

Per Serving:

calorie: 134 | fat: 3g | protein: 4g | carbs: 24g | sugars: 4g | fiber: 3g | sodium: 12mg

Mediterranean Chef Salad

Prep time: 20 minutes | Cook time: 0 minutes |

Serves 4

½ cup extra-virgin olive oil	rinsed and drained
½ cup red wine vinegar	1 medium cucumber, peeled and diced
2 tablespoons grated Parmesan cheese	½ cup diced roasted red peppers
1 teaspoon dried Italian herb blend	½ cup pitted and sliced kalamata olives
1 (15 ounces) can chickpeas,	½ cup crumbled feta cheese

4 cups spinach, romaine, and   arugula salad mix, divided

1. In large bowl, whisk together the olive oil, red wine vinegar, Parmesan cheese, and Italian herbs. 2. Add the chickpeas, cucumber, red peppers, olives, and feta cheese and mix until everything is coated well. 3. Divide the greens into 4 bowls and top each with 1 cup of the salad mix.

Per Serving:

calorie: 318 | fat: 22g | protein: 10g | carbs: 20g | sugars: 5g | fiber: 7g | sodium: 510mg

Young Kale and Cabbage Salad with Toasted Peanuts

Prep time: 15 minutes | Cook time: 0 minutes |

Serves 6

2 bunches baby kale, thinly sliced	1 teaspoon ground cumin
	¼ teaspoon smoked paprika
½ head green savoy cabbage, cored and thinly sliced	1 medium red bell pepper, thinly sliced
¼ cup apple cider vinegar	1 cup toasted peanuts
Juice of 1 lemon	1 garlic clove, thinly sliced

1. In a large salad bowl, toss the kale and cabbage together. 2. In a small bowl, to make the dressing, whisk the vinegar, lemon juice, cumin, and paprika together. 3. Pour the dressing over the greens, and gently massage with your hands. 4. Add the pepper, peanuts, and garlic, and toss to combine.

Per Serving:

calorie: 177 | fat: 12g | protein: 8g | carbs: 13g | sugars: 5g | fiber: 5g | sodium: 31mg

Strawberry-Spinach Salad

Prep time: 15 minutes | Cook time: 0 minutes |

Serves 4

½ cup extra-virgin olive oil	and sliced
¼ cup balsamic vinegar	1 cup strawberries, sliced
1 tablespoon Worcestershire sauce	1 (6 ounces) container feta cheese, crumbled
1 (10 ounces) package baby spinach	4 tablespoons bacon bits, divided
1 medium red onion, quartered	1 cup slivered almonds, divided

1. In a large bowl, whisk together the olive oil, balsamic vinegar, and Worcestershire sauce. 2. Add the spinach, onion, strawberries, and feta cheese and mix until all the ingredients are coated. 3. Portion into 4 servings and top each with 1 tablespoon of bacon bits and ¼ cup of slivered almonds.

Per Serving:

calorie: 417 | fat: 29g | protein: 24g | carbs: 19g | sugars: 7g | fiber: 7g | sodium: 542mg

Blueberry and Chicken Salad on a Bed of Greens

Prep time: 10 minutes | Cook time: 0 minutes |

Serves 4

2 cups chopped cooked chicken
1 cup fresh blueberries
¼ cup finely chopped almonds
1 celery stalk, finely chopped
¼ cup finely chopped red onion
1 tablespoon chopped fresh basil
1 tablespoon chopped fresh

cilantro
½ cup plain, nonfat Greek yogurt or vegan mayonnaise
¼ teaspoon salt
¼ teaspoon freshly ground black pepper
8 cups salad greens (baby spinach, spicy greens, romaine)

1. In a large mixing bowl, combine the chicken, blueberries, almonds, celery, onion, basil, and cilantro. Toss gently to mix. 2. In a small bowl, combine the yogurt, salt, and pepper. Add to the chicken salad and stir to combine. 3. Arrange 2 cups of salad greens on each of 4 plates and divide the chicken salad among the plates to serve.

Per Serving:
calories: 207 | fat: 6g | protein: 28g | carbs: 11g | sugars: 6g | fiber: 3g | sodium: 235mg

Triple-Berry and Jicama Spinach Salad

Prep time: 30 minutes | Cook time: 0 minutes |

Serves 6

Dressing
¼ cup fresh raspberries
3 tablespoons hot pepper jelly
2 tablespoons canola oil
2 tablespoons raspberry vinegar or red wine vinegar
2 medium jalapeño chiles, seeded, finely chopped (2 tablespoons)
2 teaspoons finely chopped shallot

¼ teaspoon salt
1 small clove garlic, crushed
Salad
1 bag (6 ounces) fresh baby spinach leaves
1 cup bite-size strips (1x¼x¼ inch) peeled jicama
1 cup fresh blackberries
1 cup fresh raspberries
1 cup sliced fresh strawberries

1 In small food processor or blender, combine all dressing ingredients; process until smooth. 2 In large bowl, toss spinach and ¼ cup of the dressing. On 6 serving plates, arrange salad. To serve, top each salad with jicama, blackberries, raspberries, strawberries and drizzle with scant 1 tablespoon of remaining dressing.

Per Serving:
calorie: 120 | fat: 5g | protein: 2g | carbs: 18g | sugars: 9g | fiber: 5g | sodium: 125mg

Sweet Beet Grain Bowl

Prep time: 10 minutes | Cook time: 20 minutes |

Serves 2

3 cups water
1 cup farro, rinsed
2 tablespoons extra-virgin olive oil
1 tablespoon honey
3 tablespoons cider vinegar
Pinch freshly ground black

pepper
4 small cooked beets, sliced
1 pear, cored and diced
6 cups mixed greens
⅓ cup pumpkin seeds, roasted
¼ cup ricotta cheese

1. In a medium saucepan, stir together the water and farro over high heat and bring to a boil. Reduce the heat to medium and simmer until the farro is tender, 15 to 20 minutes. Drain and rinse the farro under cold running water until cool. Set aside. 2. Meanwhile, in a small bowl, whisk together the extra-virgin olive oil, honey, and vinegar. Season with black pepper. 3. Evenly divide the farro between two bowls. Top each with the beets, pear, greens, pumpkin seeds, and ricotta. Drizzle the bowls with the dressing before serving and adjust the seasonings as desired.

Per Serving:
calorie: 750 | fat: 28g | protein: 21g | carbs: 104g | sugars: 18g | fiber: 12g | sodium: 174mg

First-of-the-Season Tomato, Peach, and Strawberry Salad

Prep time: 15 minutes | Cook time: 0 minutes |

Serves 6

6 cups mixed spring greens
4 large ripe plum tomatoes, thinly sliced
4 large ripe peaches, pitted and thinly sliced
12 ripe strawberries, thinly sliced

½ Vidalia onion, thinly sliced
2 tablespoons white balsamic vinegar
2 tablespoons extra-virgin olive oil
Freshly ground black pepper

1. Put the greens in a large salad bowl, and layer the tomatoes, peaches, strawberries, and onion on top. 2. Dress with the vinegar and oil, toss together, and season with pepper.

Per Serving:
calorie: 122 | fat: 5g | protein: 3g | carbs: 19g | sugars: 14g | fiber: 4g | sodium: 20mg

Chicken, Cantaloupe, Kale, and Almond Salad

Prep time: 10 minutes | Cook time: 0 minutes | Serves 3

For The Salad
4 cups chopped kale, packed
1½ cups diced cantaloupe
1½ cups shredded rotisserie chicken
½ cup sliced almonds

¼ cup crumbled feta
For The Dressing
2 teaspoons honey
2 tablespoons extra-virgin olive oil
2 teaspoons apple cider vinegar or freshly squeezed lemon juice

To Make The Salad 1. Divide the kale into three portions. Layer ⅓ of the cantaloupe, chicken, almonds, and feta on each portion. 2. Drizzle some of the dressing over each portion of salad. Serve immediately. To Make The Dressing 3. In a small bowl, whisk together the honey, olive oil, and vinegar.

Per Serving:

calorie: 376 | fat: 23g | protein: 30g | carbs: 16g | sugars: 12g | fiber: 3g | sodium: 415mg

Greek Island Potato Salad

Prep time: 5 minutes | Cook time: 35 minutes | Serves 10

⅓ cup extra-virgin olive oil
4 garlic cloves, minced
2 pounds red potatoes, cut into 1½-inch pieces (leave the skin on if you wish)
6 medium carrots, peeled, halved lengthwise, and cut into 1½-inch

pieces
1 onion, chopped
16 ounces artichoke hearts packed in water, drained and cut in half
½ cup Kalamata olives, pitted and halved
¼ cup lemon juice

1. In a large skillet, heat the olive oil. Add the garlic, and sauté for 30 seconds. Add the potatoes, carrots, and onion; cook over medium heat for 25 to 30 minutes until vegetables are just tender. 2. Add the artichoke hearts, and cook for 3 to 5 minutes more. Remove from the heat, and stir in the olives and lemon juice. Season with a dash of salt and pepper. Transfer to a serving bowl, and serve warm.

Per Serving:

calorie: 178 | fat: 8g | protein: 4g | carbs: 25g | sugars: 4g | fiber: 6g | sodium: 134mg

Appendix 1: Measurement Conversion Chart

MEASUREMENT CONVERSION CHART

VOLUME EQUIVALENTS(DRY)

US STANDARD	METRIC (APPROXIMATE)
1/8 teaspoon	0.5 mL
1/4 teaspoon	1 mL
1/2 teaspoon	2 mL
3/4 teaspoon	4 mL
1 teaspoon	5 mL
1 tablespoon	15 mL
1/4 cup	59 mL
1/2 cup	118 mL
3/4 cup	177 mL
1 cup	235 mL
2 cups	475 mL
3 cups	700 mL
4 cups	1 L

VOLUME EQUIVALENTS(LIQUID)

US STANDARD	US STANDARD (OUNCES)	METRIC (APPROXIMATE)
2 tablespoons	1 fl.oz.	30 mL
1/4 cup	2 fl.oz.	60 mL
1/2 cup	4 fl.oz.	120 mL
1 cup	8 fl.oz.	240 mL
1 1/2 cup	12 fl.oz.	355 mL
2 cups or 1 pint	16 fl.oz.	475 mL
4 cups or 1 quart	32 fl.oz.	1 L
1 gallon	128 fl.oz.	4 L

TEMPERATURES EQUIVALENTS

FAHRENHEIT(F)	CELSIUS(C) (APPROXIMATE)
225 °F	107 °C
250 °F	120 °C
275 °F	135 °C
300 °F	150 °C
325 °F	160 °C
350 °F	180 °C
375 °F	190 °C
400 °F	205 °C
425 °F	220 °C
450 °F	235 °C
475 °F	245 °C
500 °F	260 °C

WEIGHT EQUIVALENTS

US STANDARD	METRIC (APPROXIMATE)
1 ounce	28 g
2 ounces	57 g
5 ounces	142 g
10 ounces	284 g
15 ounces	425 g
16 ounces (1 pound)	455 g
1.5 pounds	680 g
2 pounds	907 g

Appendix 2: The Dirty Dozen and Clean Fifteen

The Dirty Dozen and Clean Fifteen

The Environmental Working Group (EWG) is a nonprofit, nonpartisan organization dedicated to protecting human health and the environment Its mission is to empower people to live healthier lives in a healthier environment. This organization publishes an annual list of the twelve kinds of produce, in sequence, that have the highest amount of pesticide residue-the Dirty Dozen-as well as a list of the fifteen kinds ofproduce that have the least amount of pesticide residue-the Clean Fifteen.

THE DIRTY DOZEN

- The 2016 Dirty Dozen includes the following produce. These are considered among the year's most important produce to buy organic:

Strawberries	Spinach
Apples	Tomatoes
Nectarines	Bell peppers
Peaches	Cherry tomatoes
Celery	Cucumbers
Grapes	Kale/collard greens
Cherries	Hot peppers

- *The Dirty Dozen list contains two additional itemskale/collard greens and hot peppers-because they tend to contain trace levels of highly hazardous pesticides.*

THE CLEAN FIFTEEN

- The least critical to buy organically are the Clean Fifteen list. The following are on the 2016 list:

Avocados	Papayas
Corn	Kiw
Pineapples	Eggplant
Cabbage	Honeydew
Sweet peas	Grapefruit
Onions	Cantaloupe
Asparagus	Cauliflower
Mangos	

- *Some of the sweet corn sold in the United States are made from genetically engineered (GE) seedstock. Buy organic varieties of these crops to avoid GE produce.*

Made in the USA
Las Vegas, NV
16 September 2023

77650532R00070